T0316694

Curbside
Consultation
in GI Cancer for the Gastroenterologist

49 Clinical Questions

Curbside Consultation in Gastroenterology
SERIES

SERIES EDITOR, FRANCIS A. FARRAYE, MD, MSc

Curbside
Consultation
in GI Cancer for the Gastroenterologist

49 Clinical Questions

Edited by

Douglas G. Adler, MD, FACG, AGAF, FASGE
Associate Professor of Medicine
Director of Therapeutic Endoscopy
Gastroenterology and Hepatology
University of Utah School of Medicine
Huntsman Cancer Institute
Salt Lake City, Utah

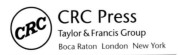

CRC Press
Taylor & Francis Group
Boca Raton London New York

CRC Press is an imprint of the
Taylor & Francis Group, an **informa** business

First published 2011 by SLACK Incorporated

Published 2024 by CRC Press
2385 NW Executive Center Drive, Suite 320, Boca Raton FL 33431

and by CRC Press
4 Park Square, Milton Park, Abingdon, Oxon, OX14 4RN

CRC Press is an imprint of Taylor & Francis Group, LLC

© 2011 Taylor & Francis Group, LLC

Library of Congress Cataloging-in-Publication Data

Curbside consultation in GI cancer for the gastroenterologist : 49 clinical questions / edited by Douglas Adler.
    p. ; cm. -- (Curbside consultation in gastroenterology)
  Includes bibliographical references and index.
  ISBN 978-1-55642-984-2 (alk. paper)
 1. Digestive organs--Cancer. I. Adler, Douglas (Douglas G.), 1969- II. Series: Curbside consultation in gastroen-terology.
  [DNLM: 1. Gastrointestinal Neoplasms--diagnosis. 2. Gastrointestinal Neoplasms--therapy. WI 149]
  RC280.D5C87 2011
  616.99'43--dc22
                              2011004848

ISBN: 9781556429842 (pbk)
ISBN: 9781003523536 (ebk)

DOI: 10.1201/9781003523536

Dedication

This book is gratefully dedicated to my children, my wife, and my parents for their endless love, support, and encouragement.

Contents

Acknowledgments

I would like to thank Dr. Francis Farraye for receiving my idea for this book so enthusiastically and for helping me turn it into a reality. I am indebted to Carrie Kotlar and Alanna Franchetti of SLACK Incorporated for their wisdom and help at every phase of development. Finally, I would also like to thank Dr. Todd H. Baron for many years of both mentorship and friendship.

About the Editor

Douglas G. Adler, MD, FACG, AGAF, FASGE received his medical degree from Cornell University Medical College. He completed his residency in internal medicine at Beth Israel Deaconess Medical Center/Harvard Medical School. Dr. Adler completed both a general GI fellowship and a therapeutic endoscopy/ERCP fellowship at Mayo Clinic in Rochester, Minnesota. He then returned to the Beth Israel Deaconess Medical Center for a fellowship in endoscopic ultrasound (EUS).

Dr. Adler is currently an Associate Professor of Medicine and Director of Therapeutic Endoscopy at the University of Utah School of Medicine in Salt Lake City, Utah. Working mostly out of the School of Medicine's Huntsman Cancer Institute, Dr. Adler's clinical, educational, and research efforts focus on the diagnosis and management of patients with gastrointestinal cancers, with an emphasis on therapeutic endoscopy. He is the author of more than 150 scientific publications and book chapters.

Contributing Authors

Harshinie C. Amaratunge, MD (Question 37)
Gastroenterology Fellow
Department of Gastroenterology and Hepatology
Baylor College of Medicine
Houston, Texas

Nikhil Banerjee, MD (Question 20)
University of Utah School of Medicine
Salt Lake City, Utah

Todd H. Baron, MD (Questions 15 and 21)
Professor of Medicine
Director of Pancreaticobiliary Endoscopy
Division of Gastroenterology and Hepatology
Mayo Clinic
Rochester, Minnesota

Devina Bhasin, MD (Question 38)
Gastoenterology and Hepatology Fellow
University Hospitals Case Medical Center
Digestive Health Insitute
Cleveland, Ohio

Allene Salcedo Burdette, MD (Questions 28 and 33)
Assistant Professor of Radiology, Medicine and Surgery
Penn State Milton S. Hershey Medical Center
Penn State Heart and Vascular Institute
Hershey, Pennsylvania

Clifford S. Cho, MD, FACS (Questions 39 and 40)
Assistant Professor
Section of Surgical Oncology
University of Wisconsin School of Medicine and Public Health
Madison, Wisconsin

David Chu, MD (Questions 19 and 42)
Department of Internal Medicine
University of Utah
Salt Lake City, Utah

Peter Darwin, MD (Question 41)
Associate Professor of Medicine
Director, GI Endoscopy
University of Maryland School of Medicine
Baltimore, Maryland

Ananya Das, MD, FACG, FASGE (Questions 5 and 29)
Director, Arizona Center for Digestive Health
Associate Editor, *Gastrointestinal Endoscopy*
Gilbert, Arizona

Christopher J. DiMaio, MD (Question 2)
Assistant Attending Physician
Gastroenterology and Nutrition Service
Memorial Sloan-Kettering Cancer Center
New York, New York

John Fang, MD (Question 6)
Associate Professor of Medicine
Division of Gastroenterology, Hepatology and Nutrition
University of Utah Health Sciences Center
Salt Lake City, Utah

Ashley L. Faulx, MD, FASGE (Questions 4 and 38)
Assistant Professor of Medicine
Case School of Medicine
Digestive Health Institute
University Hospitals Case Medical Center
Cleveland, Ohio

Leyla J. Ghazi, MD (Question 46)
Assistant Professor of Medicine
University of Maryland School of Medicine
Department of Gastroenterology and Hepatology
University of Maryland Medical Center
Baltimore, Maryland

Robert E. Glasgow, MD (Questions 9 and 13)
Section Chief, Gastrointestinal and General Surgery
Associate Professor of Surgery
Department of Surgery
University of Utah
Salt Lake City, Utah

Eric Goldberg, MD (Question 34)
Assistant Professor of Medicine
University of Maryland School of Medicine
Division of Gastroenterology
University of Maryland Medical Center
Baltimore, Maryland

Fredric D. Gordon, MD (Questions 32 and 35)
Assistant Professor of Medicine
Tufts University School of Medicine
Department of Transplantation
Lahey Clinic Medical Center
Burlington, Massachusetts

Bruce D. Greenwald, MD (Question 1)
Professor of Medicine
Division of Gastroenterology and Hepatology
Department of Medicine
University of Maryland School of Medicine and Greenebaum Cancer Center
Baltimore, Maryland

Katarina B. Greer, MD, MS (Question 4)
Gastroenterology Fellow
University Hospitals Case Medical Center
Cleveland, Ohio

Kevin D. Halsey, MD (Question 1)
Gastroenterology Fellow
Division of Gastroenterology and Hepatology
Department of Medicine
University of Maryland Medical Center
Baltimore, Maryland

William R. Hutson, MD (Questions 26 and 31)
Professor of Medicine
Director of Hepatology and Liver Transplantation
University of Utah School of Medicine
Salt Lake City, Utah

Kimberly Jones, MD (Questions 27 and 45)
Assistant Professor of Medicine
University of Utah
Department of Oncology
Huntsman Cancer Institute
Salt Lake City, Utah

Virendra Joshi, MD, AGAF (Questions 8 and 24)
Associate Professor of Medicine
Clinical Professor of Surgery
Section of Gastroenterology and Hepatology
Tulane University School of Medicine
New Orleans, Louisiana

Sergey V. Kantsevoy, MD, PhD (Questions 16 and 18)
Director of Therapeutic Endoscopy
Institute for Digestive Health and Liver Disease
Mercy Medical Center
Baltimore, Maryland

Vivek Kaul, MD, FACG (Questions 3 and 49)
Associate Professor of Medicine
Acting Chief
Division of Gastroenterology & Hepatology
URMC/Strong Memorial Hospital
Rochester, New York

Rabi Kundu, MD, FRCS (Question 25)
Director of Endoscopy
Assistant Clinical Professor of Medicine and Surgery
Director of Endoscopy
University of California San Francisco
Fresno, California

Ravinder R. Kurella, MD (Question 30)
Fellow, Gastroenterology
University of Oklahoma College of Medicine
Department of Internal Medicine
Section of Digestive Diseases
Oklahoma City, Oklahoma

Jeffrey Laczek, MD (Question 41)
Associate Professor of Medicine
Uniformed Services University of the Health Sciences
Gastroenterology Service
Tripler Army Medical Center
Honolulu, Hawaii

Robin B. Mendelsohn, MD (Question 2)
Fellow
Gastroenterology and Nutrition Service
Memorial Sloan-Kettering Cancer Center
New York, New York

James D. Morris, MD (Question 24)
Assistant Professor of Medicine
Louisiana State University Health Sciences in Shreveport
Section of Gastroenterology and Hepatology
Shreveport, Louisiana
Clinical Instructor of Medicine
Tulane University School of Medicine
New Orleans, Louisiana

Sean J. Mulvihill, MD (Question 22)
Chairman, Department of Surgery
Senior Director, Clinical Affairs
Huntsman Cancer Institute
University of Utah
Salt Lake City, Utah

Randall K. Pearson, MD (Questions 14 and 17)
Associate Professor of Medicine
Mayo Clinic College of Medicine
Division of Gastroenterology and Hepatology
Rochester, Minnesota

Douglas Pleskow, MD, AGAF, FASGE (Questions 23 and 25)
Associate Clinical Professor of Medicine
Harvard Medical School
Co-Director of Endoscopy
Beth Israel Deaconess Medical Center
Boston, Massachusetts

Scott Pollack, MD (Question 8)
Metropolitan Gastroenterology Associates
New Orleans, Louisiana
Work completed during Fellowship training:
Department of Medicine
Section of Gastroenterology and Hepatology
Tulane University School of Medicine
New Orleans, Louisiana

Darryn Potosky, MD (Question 34)
Assistant Professor of Medicine
Department of Internal Medicine
Division of Gastroenterology and Hepatology
University of Maryland School of Medicine
Baltimore, Maryland

Waqar A. Qureshi, MD (Questions 37 and 43)
Professor of Medicine
Chief of Endoscopy
Baylor College of Medicine
Houston, Texas

David A. Schwartz, MD (Questions 46 and 48)
Director, Inflammatory Bowel Disease Center
Associate Professor of Medicine
Vanderbilt University Medical Center
Nashville, Tennessee

Yasser H. Shaib, MD, MPH, FASGE (Question 43)
Associate Professor of Medicine
Baylor College of Medicine
Houston, Texas

Brad Shepherd, MD (Question 48)
Clinical Instructor
Advanced Endoscopy Fellow
Vanderbilt University Medical Center
Division of Gastroenterology, Hepatology and Nutrition
Nashville, Tennessee

Andrew Singleton, MD (Question 9)
Resident
Department of Surgery
University of Utah
Salt Lake City, Utah

Colin T. Swales, MD (Question 32)
Hepatologist
Hartford Hospital
Hartford, Connecticut

Caroline R. Tadros, MD (Questions 12 and 36)
Assistant Professor of Clinical Gastroenterology
Department of Gastroenterology
The University of Utah School of Medicine
Salt Lake City, Utah

Shyam J. Thakkar, MD (Question 23)
Assistant Professor of Medicine
Temple University School of Medicine
Director of Developmental Endoscopy
West Penn Allegheny Health System
Pittsburgh, Pennsylvania

Selvi Thirumurthi, MD, MS (Questions 7 and 44)
Assistant Professor of Medicine
Baylor College of Medicine
Division of Gastroenterology and Hepatology
Ben Taub General Hospital
Houston, Texas

William M. Tierney, MD (Question 30)
Professor of Medicine
University of Oklahoma College of Medicine
Department of Internal Medicine
Section of Digestive Diseases
Oklahoma City, Oklahoma

Jeffrey L. Tokar, MD (Questions 10 and 11)
Assistant Professor
Gastroenterology Section
Fox Chase Cancer Center
Philadelphia, Pennsylvania

Ryan C. Van Woerkom, MD (Question 47)
Medical Student
University of Utah School of Medicine
Salt Lake City, Utah
Resident Physician
Department of Internal Medicine
Oregon Health and Science University
Portland, Oregon

Michael Walker, MD (Question 6)
Resident
Division of Internal Medicine
University of Utah Health Sciences Center
Salt Lake City, Utah

Paul E. Wise, MD (Question 48)
Assistant Professor of Surgery
Director, Vanderbilt Hereditary Colorectal Cancer Registry
Vanderbilt University Medical Center
Division of General Surgery
Nashville, Tennessee

Robert C. Wrona, MD (Question 13)
Resident
Department of Surgery
University of Utah
Salt Lake City, Utah

Preface

The role of the gastroenterologist continues to evolve. With the development and widespread use of therapeutic and interventional endoscopy, gastroenterologists are being called upon with increasing frequency to care for patients with known or suspected cancer. Patients requiring tissue acquisition, biliary decompression, relief from luminal obstruction, cancer screening, and post-treatment surveillance are now commonly encountered, and modern gastroenterologists need to be equipped with the knowledge and technical expertise to manage these and other cancer-related clinical problems.

In the 49 chapters that follow, some of the most challenging and complex questions in gastrointestinal cancer care are explored in detail with an eye on useful, practical advice for clinical gastroenterologists. Key issues in the diagnosis and management of clinical problems associated with esophageal, gastric, and small and large bowel cancers are covered. Extensive space in this book is also devoted to pancreatic, biliary, and primary hepatic tumors as the rapid rise of endoscopic ultrasound (EUS) and the ongoing widespread use of endoscopic retrograde cholangiopancreatography (ERCP) have made gastroenterologists the "point of the spear" for both diagnosis and management of tumors that were in the past primarily cared for by surgeons. Additional chapters focus on important problems in the diagnosis and management of ampullary cancers, gastrointestinal stromal tumors (GISTs), hereditary cancer syndromes, screening and surveillance of colorectal cancer, anal cancer, and other relevant issues.

This book strongly endorses the multidisciplinary approach to the care of patients with gastrointestinal cancers that is employed at most major cancer centers. In addition to the chapters written by gastroenterologists, many of the individual chapters are written by general surgeons, medical and surgical oncologists, and interventional radiologists. These authors provide valuable perspective on how interlocking care from multiple physicians can result in the best outcomes for cancer patients.

The chapters in this book also frequently focus on complications—both how to avoid them and how to manage them when they arise, as, despite our best efforts, not every patient has an ideal outcome. An awareness of potential complications is the first step in their avoidance, and the risks of the techniques and technologies discussed in this book are emphasized for the reader to assist in making the best clinical choices for patients who are often acutely ill in the setting of a chronic, debilitating illness.

I am indebted to my many coauthors for their contributions; without their efforts, this project would not have been possible.

My personal passion for, and experience with, the diagnosis and management of gastrointestinal cancers spurred me to create this book. I hope that you find this volume to be a timely, relevant, practical, and overall helpful aid to your practice.

Douglas G. Adler, MD

SECTION I

ESOPHAGUS

WHAT ARE THE RISK FACTORS FOR THE DEVELOPMENT OF ESOPHAGEAL CANCER?

Kevin D. Halsey, MD and Bruce D. Greenwald, MD

It is estimated that nearly 16,500 patients (12,900 men and 3600 women) were diagnosed with esophageal cancer in 2009, with 14,500 dying from the disease.[1] This is a 460% increase in the incidence of esophageal adenocarcinoma for White men and 335% for White women since 1970. In contrast, esophageal squamous cell carcinoma is declining in incidence. In the 1960s, squamous cell carcinoma accounted for nearly 90% of esophageal malignancies. However, adenocarcinoma presently accounts for more than 60% of the new cases. Mortality associated with esophageal cancer is related to the stage of disease at presentation, with 5-year survival rates of 35% for localized disease and 3% for metastatic disease.

Barrett's esophagus (BE; specialized intestinal metaplasia of the esophagus) is the most established risk factor for developing esophageal adenocarcinoma. The lifetime risk of developing adenocarcinoma in this condition is approximately 5%, and the risk increases to 30% at 5 years for patients with BE with high-grade dysplasia. Gastroesophageal reflux disease (GERD) is the most commonly associated risk factor for BE, and studies have linked GERD to adenocarcinoma. Those with heartburn have an increased risk for adenocarcinoma compared to asymptomatic individuals with an odds ratio (OR) of nearly 8. Those with long standing (> 20 years) and severe symptoms are at substantially increased risk for adenocarcinoma with an OR of 43.5.[2] Despite numerous studies linking GERD and esophageal adenocarcinoma, up to 40% of those diagnosed with this cancer have no history of heartburn, suggesting a possible role for asymptomatic GERD as well.

Obesity and the presence of a hiatal hernia are risk factors for severe gastroesophageal reflux. Those with GERD symptoms and a hiatal hernia are at increased risk for adenocarcinoma (OR of 8.1 versus 3.6 without hernia).[3] A meta-analysis published in 2005 identified obesity (body mass index [BMI] > 25) as a risk factor for adenocarcinoma

Figure 1-1. Subtotally obstructing squamous cell esophageal cancer seen in the mid-esophagus of a 58-year-old man with a 40-year history of heavy tobacco use. (Reprinted with permission of Douglas G. Adler, MD.)

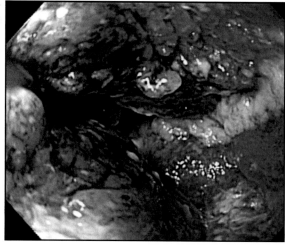

with an adjusted OR of 2.02 compared to those with a BMI less than 25. However, a separate study found that the presence of central obesity, and not solely increased BMI, was associated with an increased risk for BE.

In the United States and Western Europe, tobacco smoking and alcohol consumption are considered major risk factors for developing esophageal squamous cell carcinoma (Figure 1-1). Alcohol consumption of more than 3 drinks per day, compared to up to 1 drink daily, is associated with an increased risk with a hazard ratio (HR) of 4.93.[4] In 2007, a prospective cohort study of nearly 475,000 patients found that a current or previous history of cigarette smoking significantly increased the risk with a HR of 9.27 and 4.35, respectively.[5] Those with a history of previous oropharyngeal or hypopharyngeal carcinoma (most commonly due to tobacco exposure) are at increased risk for developing a secondary esophageal squamous cell carcinoma, with an incidence ratio (IR) of 22.76.[6]

Other conditions associated with esophageal squamous cell carcinoma are caustic ingestion (typically lye) and achalasia. Some authors estimate that caustic ingestion patients have up to a 1000-fold increased risk for esophageal squamous cell carcinoma, with cancer developing approximately 30 years after ingestion.[7] A cohort study assessing 2900 patients with achalasia found a 10-fold increase in the incidence of esophageal malignancy.[8] Interestingly, they found an equal distribution between both esophageal squamous cell carcinoma and adenocarcinoma.

A previous history of esophageal cancer is an important risk factor for recurrent malignancy. Adenocarcinoma patients treated with esophagectomy remain at an increased risk for recurrent dysplastic BE and adenocarcinoma. A recent study reported recurrent disease in 8 of 45 patients (18%) with adenocarcinoma who underwent esophagectomy with removal of all BE and malignancy. Three patients developed either high-grade dysplasia or recurrent adenocarcinoma at intervals of 7, 18, and 88 months following their surgical cure.[9] In addition, approximately 80% of patients who have completed definitive combined chemotherapy and external beam radiation for esophageal adenocarcinoma associated with BE will have persistent BE and would be expected to remain at considerable increased risk for a recurrent adenocarcinoma.

Esophageal squamous cell carcinoma patients undergoing curative surgical resection or definitive chemoradiation also remain at an increased risk for recurrent malignancy. A recent study identified an 18% locoregional recurrence rate in 171 patients undergoing extended radical esophagectomy despite achieving an overall 5-year survival rate of 55%.[10] The median disease-free interval until recurrence was 11 months. Recurrence rates for esophageal squamous cell carcinoma patients treated with either definitive chemoradiation therapy or local endoscopic resection are likely higher.

Cost-efficient and cost-effective endoscopic screening programs are essential in reducing the burden of esophageal cancer. There are no specific consensus guidelines indicating who and when to screen for esophageal squamous cell carcinoma, and tobacco and alcohol use remains widespread. Recently published consensus guidelines discussed the difficulties involving the implementation of screening programs for esophageal adenocarcinoma. The authors concluded that inadequate data preclude general screening and screening in higher risk groups, such as White men older than 50 years with longstanding heartburn, should be individualized. However, as previously mentioned, up to 40% of patients diagnosed with esophageal adenocarcinoma have no previous history of heartburn. In addition, sampling error associated with screening biopsies decreases the efficiency of screening programs in patients with BE. Standard 4-quadrant biopsy protocols are imperfect, time-consuming, and not universally performed. Targeted biopsies theoretically decrease sampling error and improve time efficiency. Lugol's iodine solution has a high affinity for glycogen in nonkeratinized squamous epithelium and is used for chromoendoscopic screening in patients at risk for esophageal squamous cell carcinoma. Several new technologies are being evaluated for targeted biopsies in BE, including high-definition endoscopic imaging in combination with narrow-band or multi-band imaging.

The impact of these techniques on clinical outcomes has not been established in large trials, but will likely serve to improve visualization and will hopefully facilitate better targeting of biopsies to enhance screening efforts.

References

1. Horner MJ, Ries LAG, Krapcho M, et al. *SEER Cancer Statistics Review, 1975-2006,* National Cancer Institute. Bethesda, MD. http://seer.cancer.gov/csr/1975_2006/, based on November 2008 SEER data submission, posted to the SEER web site, 2009. Accessed March 20, 2010.
2. Lagergren J, Bergstrom R, Lindgren A, Nyren O. Symptomatic gastroesophageal reflux as a risk factor for esophageal adenocarcinoma. *N Engl J Med.* 1999;340(11):825-831.
3. Wu AH, Tseng CC, Bernstein L. Hiatal hernia, reflux symptoms, body size, and risk of esophageal and gastric adenocarcinoma. *Cancer.* 2003;98(5):940-948.
4. Anderson LA, Cantwell MM, Peter Watson RG, et al. The association between alcohol and reflux esophagitis, Barrett's esophagus, and esophageal adenocarcinoma. *Gastroenterology.* 2009;136(3):799-805.
5. Freedman ND, Abnet CC, Leitzmann MF, et al. A prospective study of tobacco, alcohol, and the risk of esophageal and gastric subtypes. *Am J Epidemiol.* 2007;165(12):1424-1433.
6. Lee KD, Chen PT, Chan CH, et al. The incidence and risk of developing a second primary esophageal cancer in patients with oral and pharyngeal carcinoma: a population-based study in Taiwan over a 25 year period. *BMC Cancer.* 2009;9:373.
7. Kochhar R, Sethy PK, Kochhar S, Nagi B, Gupta NM. Corrosive induced carcinoma of esophagus: report of three patients and review of literature. *J Gastroenterol Hepatol.* 2006;21(4):777-780.
8. Zendehdel K, Nyren O, Edberg A, Ye W. Risk of esophageal adenocarcinoma in achalasia patients, a retrospective cohort study in Sweden. *Am J Gastroenterol.* 2007;102:1-5.

9. Wolfsen HC, Hemminger LL, DeVault KR. Recurrent Barrett's esophagus and adenocarcinoma after esophagectomy. *BMC Gastroenterol.* 2004;4:18.
10. Nakagawa S, Kanda T, Kosugi S, Ohashi M, Suzuki T, Hatakeyama K. Recurrence pattern of squamous cell carcinoma of the thoracic esophagus after extended radical esophagectomy with three-field lymphadenectomy. *J Am Coll Surg.* 2004;198(2):205-211.

DO ALL PATIENTS WITH ESOPHAGEAL CANCER REQUIRE SURGERY OR CAN SOME BE MANAGED WITH NONSURGICAL (ENDOSCOPIC, ONCOLOGIC, ETC) METHODS ALONE?

Robin B. Mendelsohn, MD and Christopher J. DiMaio, MD

The incidence of esophageal cancer has increased in recent years. The American Cancer Society estimates that there will be 16,640 new cases and 14,500 deaths from esophageal cancer in the United States in 2010.[1] Though it is a relatively rare cancer, it is an aggressive and lethal cancer with an overall 5-year survival rate ranging from 5% to 50%.

The diagnosis of esophageal cancer is usually confirmed by endoscopy with biopsy. There are 2 main types of esophageal cancer: adenocarcinoma (AC), which is often associated with gastroesophageal reflux disease and Barrett's esophagus (BE), and squamous cell carcinoma (SCC), which is often associated with tobacco and alcohol use. Other rare types include small cell carcinoma, leiomyosarcoma, lymphoma, and gastrointestinal stromal tumor (GIST).

Once you have made the diagnosis, the next step is to attempt to stage the tumor to determine the extent of involvement of the esophageal wall as well as to evaluate whether the tumor has spread to local tissues or other organs. Though there is debate as to which tests to use, most experts advocate computed tomography (CT) of the chest and abdomen to assess for local and distant metastasis and endoscopic ultrasound (EUS) to assess degree of tumor invasion in the esophageal wall and to evaluate for the presence or absence of regional lymph node involvement. This strategy gives the most accurate overall staging information.

Figure 2-1. EMR removal of a stage I esophageal cancer using a fitted cap device. The lesion is brought into the cap and removed with a hot snare. Resection in this case was complete.

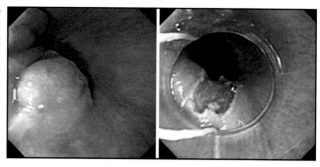

You can then individualize treatment options based on disease histology, disease stage, patient comorbidities, and patient preference. Options include surgery, endoscopic therapies, chemotherapy, radiation, or a combination thereof. Traditionally, surgery was the mainstay of treatment for cure and palliation. Esophagectomy, however, has low cure rates and is associated with significant morbidity and mortality even in expert hands. Therefore, many are moving toward a multidisciplinary approach in an attempt to provide patients with more options in a controlled and semi-standardized manner.

Surgery remains the standard of care for early stage cancers (stage I, tumor invades lamina propria or submucosa). The alternative options to surgery include endoscopic mucosal resection (EMR), EMR followed by chemoradiotherapy, endoscopic ablative techniques, and definitive chemotherapy, radiation, or combined chemoradiation.

EMR is a technique whereby the target lesion is lifted away from the submucosa by either using a submucosal fluid injection or by raising the lesion with a cap or band-assistive device. The target lesion is then removed with a hot snare (Figure 2-1).

EMR was first described in the esophagus by Mukuuchi in Japan in 1988 and has been adopted by Western centers during the past 2 decades. There are 2 main characteristics that make a lesion amenable to EMR. The first is that it does not infiltrate the deep layers of the esophageal wall. This is based on surgical data that demonstrated that patients who underwent curative surgeries for early stage esophageal cancers had virtually no or minimal risk of metastasis if the lesion was confined to the mucosa or lamina propria, a 10% risk if the lesion reached the muscularis mucosa or the upper submucosa, and up to 50% risk if the lesion showed deep invasion of the submucosa. Therefore, only mucosal lesions are usually considered for EMR for potential of cure. That being said, submucosal lesions can be technically removed by EMR and may be considered in patients who refuse surgery or who are not surgical candidates, with the understanding that those lesions carry a higher risk of metastasis. The second characteristic is that the lesion should not exceed two-thirds of the circumference of the esophagus. This is because circumferential mucosal resection carries a risk of post-procedure stricture formation. Most of the studies of EMR were performed in Japan with SCC and demonstrated at least comparable outcomes to surgery with much less morbidity and virtually no mortality. Though the data for EMR with AC are more limited, there is emerging evidence that this technique has similar outcomes to the SCC group.[2,3]

A second nonsurgical option is EMR followed by prophylactic chemoradiation for possible lymph node metastasis. This can be considered in patients whose lesions invade the muscularis mucosa or the upper submucosa because, as mentioned above, these patients have a higher risk of lymph node metastasis. There are currently prospective trials going on to further investigate this approach. To date, this has only been studied in SCC.

A third option is endoscopic ablation via either cryoablation, radiofrequency ablation (RFA), or photodynamic therapy (PDT). Cryoablation involves spraying liquid nitrogen at low pressure though an endoscopic catheter. Preliminary data show that this is safe and effective for the eradication of BE and early esophageal cancers. Further long-term studies are needed.[4] Similarly, RFA employs the use of specially designed balloons and catheters to allow targeted delivery of ablative energy to the tumor. Again, early studies are promising, but further data are needed.[5] Photodynamic therapy uses photosensitizing agents, laser light, and reactive oxygen species to endoscopically destroy the cancer cells. PDT has been proven effecive and actually provides the deepest tissue destruction of the ablative therapies, but has fallen out of favor due to a relatively high complication rate, most notably photosensitivity-related skin burns and postprocedure strictures.

Definitive chemoradiation is also an option. Studies out of Japan have shown excellent response and survival rates for patients with stage II SCC receiving 5-fluorouracil (5-FU) and cisplatin and concurrently receiving external beam radiation. Similarly, a randomized study done in the United States (RTOG 85-01) looked at patients with SCC or AC and randomized them to chemotherapy with 5-FU and cisplatin and radiation, or radiation alone, and found a significant improvement in both median survival and 5-year survival in the combination group.[6] This study included patients with stage I to III cancers, but found a significant benefit in all 3 stages.

For stage II and III disease (tumor invading beyond the muscularis propria, with regional lymph node metastasis), definitive chemoradiotherapy remains the most commonly employed nonsurgical option based on the RTOG study described previously (Figure 2-2). In the past, many patients who responded to neoadjuvant chemoradiation went on to esophagectomy. Increasing evidence shows that chemoradiation alone may produce equivalent results.[7,8]

For patients with stage IV disease (distant metastasis), most treatments are palliative interventions for dysphagia, bleeding, and pain control. Endoscopic modalities for dysphagia include laser therapy, balloon dilation, and placement of self-expanding metal stents (Figure 2-3). In some cases, placement of percutaneous endoscopic gastrostomy or jejunostomy tubes may be necessary for adequate nutrition. Radiation, chemotherapy, and combined chemotherapy have been used for palliation of both dysphagia and bleeding.

Conclusion

Esophageal cancer can be managed with nonsurgical methods including endoscopy, chemotherapy, radiation, or a combination of modalities. Treatment should be individualized, based on the stage of the cancer, patient comorbidities, and patient preference.

Figure 2-2A. Pretreatment endoscopic images of a patient with locally advanced esophageal adenocarcinoma involving the cardia of the stomach as well.

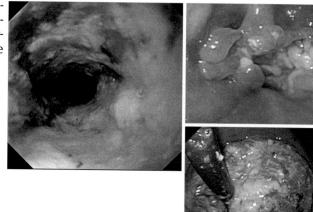

Figure 2-2B. Endoscopic images of the same patient following chemoradiation therapy showing marked improvement.

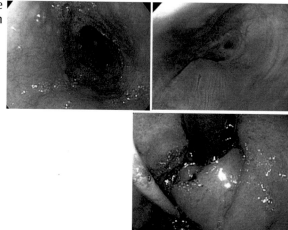

Figure 2-3. Stage IV esophageal cancer treated via a self-expanding metal stent.

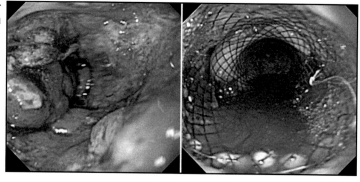

References

1. American Cancer Society. *Cancer Facts & Figures 2010.* Atlanta, GA: American Cancer Society; 2010.
2. Inoue H, Fukami N, Yoshida T, et al. Endoscopic mucosal resection for esophageal and gastric cancers. *J Gastroenterol Hepatol.* 2002;17(4):382-388.
3. Ciocirlan N, Lapalus MG, Hervieu V, et al. Endoscopic mucosal resection for squamous premalignant and early malignant lesions of the esophagus. *Endoscopy.* 2007;39(1):24-29.
4. Greenwald BD, Dumot JA, Abrams JA, et al. Endoscopic spray cryotherapy for esophageal cancer: safety and efficacy. *Gastrointest Endosc.* 2010;71(4):686-693.
5. Zhang YM, Bergman JJ, Weusten B, et al. Radiofrequency ablation for early esophageal squamous neoplasia. *Endoscopy.* 2010;42(4):327-333.
6. Cooper JS, Guo MD, Hersovic AM, et al. Chemoradiotherapy of locally advanced esophageal cancer: long-term follow-up of a prospective randomized trial (RTOG 85-01). Radiation Therapy Oncology Group. *JAMA.* 1999;281(17):1623-1627.
7. Bedenne L, Michel P, Bouché O, et al. Chemoradiation followed by surgery compared with chemoradiation alone in squamous cancer of the esophagus: FFCD 9102. *J Clin Oncol.* 2007;25(10):1160-1168.
8. Gebski V, Burmeister B, Smithers BM, et al. Survival benefits from neoadjuvant chemoradiotherapy or chemotherapy in oesophageal carcinoma: a meta-analysis. *Lancet Oncol.* 2007;8(3):226-234.

WHAT OPTIONS EXIST FOR ENTERAL FEEDING IN PREOPERATIVE PATIENTS WITH ESOPHAGEAL CANCER WHO HAVE DYSPHAGIA?

Vivek Kaul, MD, FACG

In patients with esophageal cancer, dysphagia presents an additional unique nutritional challenge (beyond anorexia and tumor-related cachexia). As is frequently the case, the majority of patients who present with dysphagia are found to have significant esophageal luminal obstruction at the time of diagnosis. Baseline nutritional status is an independent predictive factor for treatment response and survival in these patients.[1] Malnutrition is associated with increased perioperative morbidity and prolonged hospital stay. For this reason, nutritional support should be addressed as a high priority in these patients.

A critical aspect of the management of preoperative patients with esophageal cancer is the ability to maintain adequate nutrition and fluid intake, especially in patients who undergo neoadjuvant therapy and/or prepare for surgery. As a significant number of patients will receive neoadjuvant therapy, an adequate means of delivering nutrition, medications, and hydration that will likely be in place for 2 to 3 months must be employed (Figure 3-1). The enteral route is preferred (over parenteral) given a functioning gut, lower complication rates, and less cost. This chapter will review the strategies for maintaining nutrition in preoperative patients with esophageal cancer and associated malignant dysphagia.

Nasoenteric Feeding Tubes

Placement of a nasoenteric feeding tube represents the easiest, quickest, and least invasive method to initiate nutritional therapy in patients with significant esophageal obstruction and malnutrition. However, most patients find it uncomfortable, the tube itself may cause sinusitis, and it is at best a temporary solution.

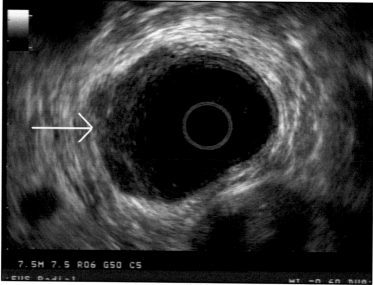

Figure 3-1. A 7.5-MHz EUS image of an esophageal adenocarcinoma. The patient's tumor has obliterated and extended completely through the muscularis propria into the adventitia, consistent with T3 disease (arrow). The patient will therefore require neoadjuvant therapy prior to surgery. (Reprinted with permission of Douglas G. Adler, MD.)

Feeding Gastrostomy Tube

A well-accepted modality to facilitate nutrition in these patients is the placement of a feeding gastrostomy tube. This can be done endoscopically (percutaneous endoscopic gastrostomy [PEG]), radiologically, or surgically. Most endoscopic PEG tubes are placed under conscious sedation as an outpatient, and feeding can usually start the next morning. The technical aspects of placing a PEG and the overall complication rates in esophageal cancer patients compare favorably with other patient populations in which PEG is placed.[2] Potential complications include procedure-related bleeding, visceral organ trauma, infection, leakage, and tube migration. PEG-related complications may compromise the immediate treatment plan. The PEG tube can remain in place for the entire duration of treatment. It can be removed easily at the bedside when no longer needed. Data on preoperative PEG tubes are mixed; some surgical oncologists are opposed to PEG tubes in preoperative patients, citing a desire not to fix the stomach to the anterior abdominal wall since the stomach needs to be mobilized proximally during surgery; other surgeons do not express this concern.[2] Although tumor seeding of the gastric wall has been reported, it is an infrequent phenomenon in larger series.[2-4]

Feeding Jejunostomy Tube

A jejunal feeding tube may be considered in some patients with esophageal cancer (known gastroparesis, prior gastric surgery/resection, etc). This can be performed endoscopically (percutaneous endoscopic jejunostomy [PEJ]), radiologically, or surgically. A jejunal tube allows more continuous feeding and potentially reduces reflux and

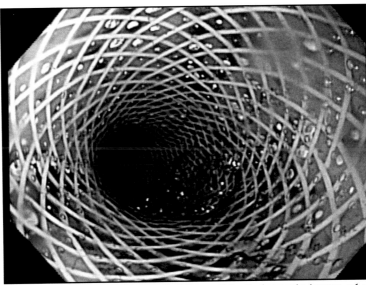

Figure 3-2. Same patient as in Figure 3-1. Endoscopic image of a self-expanding plastic stent (SEPS) placed across the tumor to palliate malignant dysphagia during neoadjuvant therapy. (Reprinted with permission of Douglas G. Adler, MD.)

associated aspiration risks. The technique of direct endoscopic jejunostomy has been well-described, although complication rates are higher and should be reserved for patients in whom PEG is not feasible.[5] Another option is a jejunal extension tube through a PEG tube (the so-called G-J tube).

Esophageal Stents

In recent years, there has been significant progress in the design, development, and application of esophageal stents for the palliation of malignant dysphagia in patients with advanced esophageal cancer or as a "bridge" to surgery, enabling improved nutritional delivery and quality of life (Figure 3-2). In the past, preoperative stenting was considered to be contraindicated, but the thinking in this area has changed dramatically in the past few years given the availability of removable, fully covered stents. Gastroenterologists and surgeons now have a wide variety of esophageal stents to choose from based on material (plastic versus metal), covering (partially or fully), removability, deployment characteristics, radial force, and a wide range of luminal diameters and lengths.[6,7]

A recent report described the successful use of the Polyflex "removable" stent (Boston Scientific, Natick, MA) for palliation of malignant dysphagia in patients undergoing neoadjuvant therapy, with a high level of success and no interference with neoadjuvant therapy or surgery[8] (Figure 3-2). Fully covered ("removable") esophageal self-expandable metal stents (SEMS) have also become available from several manufacturers in the past few years. Published data on these devices are limited, and their role in malignant esophageal obstruction needs further clarification, but they are likely to play a growing role in preoperative patients with esophageal cancer. Smaller-profile esophageal SEMS are being introduced to allow more customized endotherapy for very high-grade and proximal neoplastic strictures in the esophagus.

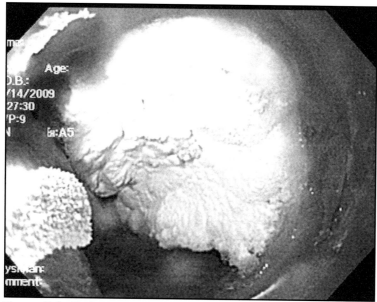

Figure 3-3. Endoscopic image of endoluminal spray cryotherapy being used to locally ablate tumor tissue in the esophagus.

Complications of stenting include chest pain, hiccoughs, nausea, vomiting, gastro-esophageal reflux disease (GERD), stent migration, bleeding, and stent occlusion secondary to food or tumor ingrowth. More serious complications, such as perforation and fistula formation (esophago-respiratory or esophago-aortic), are encountered much less frequently.

The decision to proceed with esophageal stenting should be made as part of a multidisciplinary approach toward the management of the patient with esophageal cancer. The choice of stent should be individualized to the specific goals in a particular patient. The patient should be counseled regarding the potential for stent-related complications and their management. The importance of compliance with an appropriate diet (low residue, small bites, frequent fluids, etc) in the post-stenting period cannot be overemphasized.

Endoscopic Ablative Therapies

Endoscopic "debulking" or ablation of the luminal tumor mass preoperatively can be performed using argon plasma coagulation, photodynamic therapy (PDT), Nd:YAG-laser, and endoluminal cryospray therapy.[9] Cryospray represents a novel tool for endoluminal ablation in esophageal cancer patients, given its efficacy and safety profile (Figure 3-3). However, the limited availability of this technology, the need for multiple procedures, and relatively longer time needed to achieve luminal patency (eg, compared to self-expanding metal stents) may be limiting factors in patients with severe dysphagia and malnutrition.

The goal of endoscopic ablation is to re-establish luminal patency and improve oral intake, nutritional status, and quality of life without the need for feeding tubes or esophageal stents. Occlusion of SEMS by tumor ingrowth can also be managed by endoscopic ablation, thereby restoring luminal patency and the ability to consume food orally.

Conclusion

Patients with esophageal cancer are at risk for severe malnutrition, which can impact their response to treatment and overall survival. Multiple strategies are available to help optimize the nutritional status in these patients and to achieve the best multimodal treatment results. There are pros and cons to every applicable modality aimed at improving enteral nutrition in patients with esophageal cancer. Proper discussion and informed consent is critical prior to selecting a particular intervention in a given patient. The specific approach should be individualized in each patient, after a thorough review of each modality and depending on the available local expertise, treatment goals, and multidisciplinary team recommendations, to achieve the best results.

References

1. Di Fiore F, Lecleire S, Pop D, et al. Baseline nutritional status is predictive of response to treatment and survival in patients treated by definitive chemoradiotherapy for a locally advanced esophageal cancer. *Am J Gastroenterol.* 2007;102(11):2557-2563.
2. Margolis M, Alexander P, Trachiotis GD, Gharagozloo F, Lipman T. Percutaneous endoscopic gastrostomy before multimodality therapy in patients with esophageal cancer. *Ann Thorac Surg.* 2003;76(5):1694-1698.
3. Becker G, Hess CF, Grund KE, Hoffmann W, Bamberg M. Abdominal wall metastasis following percutaneous endoscopic gastrostomy. *Support Care Cancer.* 1995;3(5):313-316.
4. Peghini PL, Guaouguaou N, Salcedo JA, Al-Kawas FH. Implantation metastasis after PEG: case report and review. *Gastrointest Endosc.* 2000;51(4):480-482.
5. Maple JT, Petersen BT, Baron TH, Gostout CJ, Wong Kee Song LM, Buttar N. Direct percutaneous endoscopic jejunostomy: Outcomes in 307 consecutive attempts. *Am J Gastroenterol.* 2005;100(12):2681-2688.
6. Siddiqui A, Loren D, Dudnick R, Kowalski T. Expandable polyester silicone-covered stent for malignant esophageal strictures before neoadjuvant chemoradiation: a pilot study. *Dig Dis Sci.* 2007;52(3):823-829.
7. Mougey A, Adler DG. Esophageal stenting for the palliation of malignant dysphagia. *J Support Oncol.* 2008;6(6):267-273.
8. Adler DG, Fang J, Wong R, Wills J, Hilden K. Placement of Polyflex stents in patients with locally advanced esophageal cancer is safe and improves dysphagia during neoadjuvant therapy. *Gastrointest Endosc.* 2009;70(4):614-619.
9. Greenwald BD, Dumot JA, Abrams JA, et al. Endoscopic spray cryotherapy for esophageal cancer: safety and efficacy. *Gastrointest Endosc.* 2010;71(4):686-693.

AN 81-YEAR-OLD MAN IS FOUND TO HAVE UNRESECTABLE ESOPHAGEAL CANCER AND MALIGNANT DYSPHAGIA. SHOULD HE HAVE A STENT? A NASOGASTRIC FEEDING TUBE? A PERCUTANEOUS ENDOSCOPIC GASTROSTOMY TUBE?

Katarina B. Greer, MD, MS and Ashley L. Faulx, MD, FASGE

Five-year survival of patients with esophageal cancer remains poor and generally does not exceed 20%. More than 50% of patients with esophageal cancer present with metastatic disease. A recent Cochrane Review based on 2 randomized controlled trials did not demonstrate any survival advantage for chemotherapy versus best supportive care in metastatic esophageal cancer.[1] The management of malignant dysphagia is thus an important goal of palliative therapy. Treatment options for dysphagia include endoscopic stenting, feeding tube placement, radiation therapy, brachytherapy, or laser treatment.

We frequently offer our patients esophageal stenting, which can restore oral intake, decrease regurgitation, prevent aspiration of retained food contents, and allow patients to enjoy some degree of oral intake. Self-expandable metal stents (SEMS) are preferred in the management of malignant dysphagia. Self-expandable plastic stents (SEPS) are equally effective in palliating dysphagia; however, they are associated with a higher rate of complications such as hemorrhage, migration, or food impaction. The delivery system for the only SEPS presently available in the United States is of a large diameter (12 to 14 mm), is somewhat stiff, and requires assembly. Fully-covered or partially-covered esophageal SEMS tend to have less tumor ingrowth compared to uncovered SEMS, although uncovered SEMS are rarely used in modern clinical practice (Figure 4-1). Most currently available stents provide comparable dysphagia relief and have similar migration rates.

Figure 4-1. An endoscopic image of an Alimaxx-E (Merit Medical Systems, Inc., South Jordan, Utah) fully covered esophageal stent in a patient with esophageal cancer. (Reprinted with permission of Douglas G. Adler, MD.)

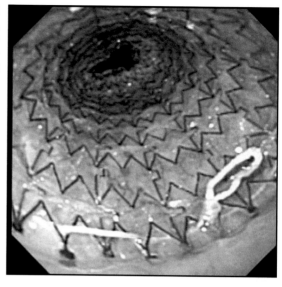

The location of the esophageal tumor is an important consideration prior to placement of an esophageal stent. Stents placed in proximity of the upper esophageal sphincter are often poorly tolerated due to pain and globus sensation. It is frequently recommended that a distance of 2 cm from the upper esophageal sphincter be maintained to minimize these symptoms. Tumors close to the gastroesophageal junction (GEJ) may not be amenable to stenting due to the fact that the stent does not have a distal tissue "shelf" against which it can be anchored. If the stent is placed such that it crosses the GEJ, it is important to tell the patient that he or she may have problems with acid reflux as gastric contents can freely return into the esophagus. We place all of these patients on high-dose proton pump inhibitors (PPIs) and ask them to elevate the head of the bed to 30 degrees and remain upright for 30 to 60 minutes after eating. Antireflux stents are available but cannot be universally advocated.[2]

Immediate complications of stent placement include perforation, aspiration, airway compromise, incorrect position, delivery system entrapment, or stent dislodgement. Bleeding, chest pain, and nausea can occur up to 1 week after stent placement, although many patients have some degree of pain immediately following stent placement. Late complications include recurrent dysphagia due to tumor ingrowth or overgrowth, food impaction, stent migration, tracheoesophageal fistula formation, bleeding, reflux, and/or aspiration. Complications from stent placement are frequent and occur in 30% to 50% of patients. Rates of complication depend on tumor location, the degree of vascularity of the obstructing lesion, prior use of chemotherapy and/or radiation therapy, stent diameter, and intrinsic stent characteristics. Larger-diameter stents generally cause more complications but are less likely to migrate, whereas narrower caliber stents tend to be better tolerated but come with an increased risk of migration. Stent placement should, in general, be performed by experienced advanced endoscopists.

A large variety of SEMS are available on the US market. Only minor differences exist between various metal stent types. Based on current evidence, routine use of a particular stent brand or type cannot be recommended. Most endoscopists typically choose stents based on personal experience combined with patient factors, such as tumor type, location, and size. As delivery systems improve, this may also influence stent choice.

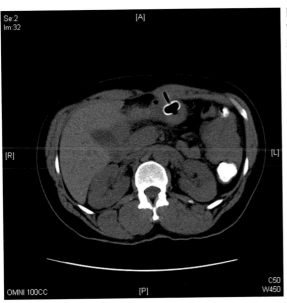

Figure 4-2. CT scan image of a PEG tube with the bumper and tube visible in the gastric lumen in a patient with unresectable esophageal cancer. (Reprinted with permission of Douglas G. Adler, MD.)

Patients with unresectable esophageal cancer and dysphagia not amenable or agreeable to stenting can benefit from percutaneous gastrostomy tube placement for nutrition support (Figure 4-2). Gastrostomy tubes can be placed by endoscopy, radiology, or surgery. Gastrostomy tubes can be used as a nutrition bridge for patients receiving chemotherapy with a reasonable expectation of response or in whom the natural history of the untreated tumor is of protracted nature and survival is expected to be greater than 6 months. Studies report up to 87% success rate of percutaneous endoscopic gastrostomy (PEG) placement, even in patients with highly obstructive lesions. Retrospective data series show some improvement in nutrition indices (albumin and prealbumin); however, they do not suggest any survival advantage in patients who choose PEG placement.[3] The most common complications of PEG placement include infection, persistent leakage, minor skin irritation, or erythema. There have been a few rare cases of tumor implantation and tract seeding with PEG placement.[4] This infrequent complication would demonstrate itself as skin changes or tissue growth around the PEG site. Tumor seeding could be prevented by PEG tube placement via radiology or surgery or via endoscopy through a Russell introducer technique, as opposed to the standard push/pull method.

Routine placement of nasogastric (NG) tubes is generally not performed. NG tubes are uncomfortable, increase the risk of sinus infection skin breakdown, and do not provide a well-tolerated means of long-term feeding access. Directed endoscopic placement of small-caliber feeding tubes secured with a bridle device may be an alternative for patients who refuse PEG or stent placement and have a short life expectancy but still need enteral access.

Ultimately, the management of malignant dysphagia in patients with advanced esophageal cancer requires constructive dialogue between the patient and physician. We feel that it is our responsibility to present our patients with information that offers best estimates of procedural success as well as complications. Thoughtful consideration of patient preference and overall health condition help finalize our treatment approach. If a patient's wish is to maintain the comforts of oral intake, he or she may opt for endoscopic stenting. Patients not amenable to stenting can still derive benefits of enteric feeding though PEG placement.

References

1. Homs MY, Gaast A, Siersema PD, Steyerberg EW, Kuipers EJ. Chemotherapy for metastatic carcinoma of the esophagus and gastroesophageal junction. *Cochrane Database Syst Rev.* 2006;4:CD004063.
2. Sharma P, Kozarek R, and the Practice Committee of the American College of Gastroenterology. Role of esophageal stents in benign and malignant diseases. *Am J Gastroenterol.* 2010;105(2):258-273.
3. Margolis M, Alexander P, Trachiotis G, Gharagozloo F, Lipman T. Percutaneous gastrostomy tube placement before multimodality therapy in patients with esophageal cancer. *Ann Thorac Surg.* 2003;76(5):1694-1698.
4. Kawasaki N, Suzuki Y, Kato T, Tsuboi K, Matsumoto A, Kashiwagi H. Metastatic hypopharyngeal and esophageal cancer to a percutaneous endoscopic gastrostomy site. *Esophagus.* 2008;5(3):155-156.

HOW SHOULD MALIGNANT TRACHEOESOPHAGEAL FISTULAE BE MANAGED IN PATIENTS WITH ESOPHAGEAL CANCER?

Ananya Das, MD, FACG, FASGE

A tracheoesophageal fistula develops in approximately 1% to 22% of all patients with esophageal cancer. These are usually caused by invasion into the respiratory tract by the malignant tumor arising from the esophagus. Although tracheal invasion is most common (50% to 60%), the fistulous communication often is with the bronchi (30% to 40%) or may be even with the peripheral lung parenchyma (3% to 10%), thus esophago-respiratory fistula (ERF) may be a more anatomically appropriate term. Generally, the fistulous communication is the end-result of a bulky aggressive tumor invading into the respiratory tract; however, it could often be the result of prior treatment such as chemotherapy, radiotherapy, photodynamic therapy, laser therapy, or even pressure necrosis related to a previously placed self-expanding metal stent (SEMS). ERF can also be seen in patients with primary lung cancer, but this only occurs in approximately 1% of cases.

The diagnosis of tracheoesophageal fistula may be difficult to make. Whenever I consult on a patient with advanced esophageal tumor, I always make a point to ask directed questions to elicit a history of repeated coughing associated with eating, drinking, or both, with a concomitant increase in dysphagia and dyspnea. Such a history is highly suggestive of the presence of an ERF. During upper endoscopy, a tracheoesophageal fistula may be clearly visible or may be difficult to detect even with a careful examination. Overall, upper endoscopy is often not very sensitive for identifying small ERFs. Contrast esophagogram with iodine-based water-soluble radiographic contrast media is useful in demonstrating a fistula if present, but should be done carefully because, if aspirated, this medium may cause bronchial irritation and pulmonary edema. Barium is the preferred contrast media in this setting because it is much better tolerated in the event of aspiration. Thoracic computed tomography (CT) is also useful as it allows one to diagnose a fistula if present but also can be used to assess the degree and severity of any concomitant aspiration pneumonitis and to plan treatment options. I find reconstructed CT images to be very useful to assess the distance of the fistula from the vocal cords and the carina in order to estimate the length of the SEMS that will be needed to seal the fistula.

Attempts should always be made to try to effectively close the fistulous opening quickly, given that ERFs markedly affect the quality of life of these patients. An untreated ERF is uniformly fatal with a median survival of only about 3 weeks. Although surgical interventions are available and have been reported to close these fistulas, in most patients, surgery is not a practical consideration due to their poor baseline functional status. Chemotherapy or radiation therapy is not helpful; often, therapy only ends up enlarging the fistulous communication. Although initial experience with rigid plastic stents was poor, the availability of partially and fully covered SEMS has revolutionized the management of tracheoesophageal fistula.

Controlled studies have shown that covered SEMS are the treatment of choice when a fistula is present or suspected. Several covered esophageal SEMS are marketed in the United States, and there have not been any studies to compare outcomes achieved with different stents. Careful assessment of the anatomy of the fistula and airway patency is needed to decide if esophageal, tracheal, or both types of stents are indicated to seal the fistula. It is often helpful to review the available imaging studies with a pulmonologist and to consider a joint procedure or separate, sequential procedures. Generally, if a tight esophageal stricture is associated with the fistula but there is no or minimal airway stenosis, then esophageal stenting with a covered SEMS alone should suffice. On the other hand, if there is no or minimal esophageal stricture, as is often seen with recurrent tumor following an Ivor-Lewis esophagectomy, an esophageal SEMS may not be effective because of the high probability of migration, and a tracheal stent may be more apt, especially in the setting of airway stenosis. Indeed, if both the esophagus and the trachea do not have significant strictures and the fistula is the main problem, then a tracheal stent may be a better option because of the lesser risk of migration. If the lumens of both the esophagus and trachea are significantly compromised by the tumor, both esophageal and tracheal stent placement will be indicated. In such a situation, both stents can be placed during a single procedure but the airway stent should be placed first because as the esophageal SEMS expands, it may compress on the trachea and convert a subclinical airway compromise into a critical narrowing.

I typically perform SEMS placement for fistula closure as an outpatient procedure with conscious sedation. However, if there is any concern for postprocedure complications such as perforation or airway compromise, the patient may need inpatient observation. I typically perform a thin-barium esophagogram a few days after covered SEMS placement to confirm sealing of the fistula (Figure 5-1). It is very important to emphasize to the patient and caregivers the steps required to avoid food impaction. These typically involve paying close attention to dentition, the consistency of ingested food, and the need for adequate chewing of each bite after SEMS placement. Food impaction often leads to a life-threatening reopening of the fistula after initial closure. If there is recurrence of symptoms such as worsening dysphagia and/or recurrent aspiration, a repeat esophagogram should be performed.

Despite the successes often seen with airway and/or esophageal stenting, complications such as perforation, hemorrhage, and recurrence of the fistula are common. In the largest reported series of SEMS placement in 61 patients with ERF, recurrence of fistula

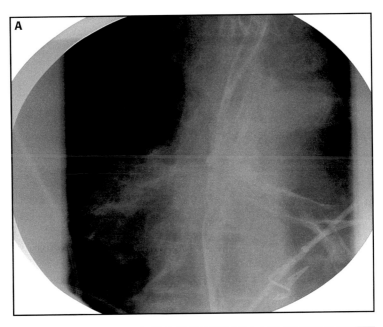

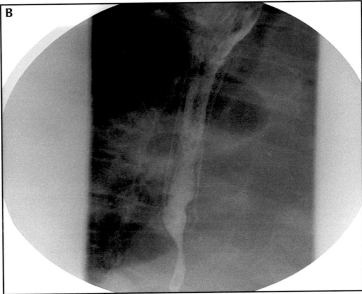

Figure 5-1. (A) Barium esophagogram with the contrast outlining the bronchial tree confirming the presence of the tracheoesophageal fistula. (B) Barium esophagogram demonstrating closure of the fistula after placement of a covered SEMS.

was encountered in up to one-third of patients after initial successful closure of the fistula over a mean follow-up period of 4.8 weeks.[1] Incomplete initial closure of the fistula occurs in up to 20% of patients and is often due to a "funnel phenomenon," which occurs due to spillage of material through a gap between the stent and the esophageal wall. Placement of a second covered SEMS through the initially placed SEMS may be helpful. A second SEMS placement may also be indicated in cases of stent occlusion due to tumor ingrowth or overgrowth.

Overall, reported success rates of initial fistula closure with covered SEMS placement range from 70% to 100% with associated complication rates of 10% to 30%.[2] Initial fistula closure is achieved in 80% of cases, and the overall mean survival in these patients is approximately 12 weeks; however, it is significantly longer in those with complete closure of the fistula.[1] Given the paucity of alternative management options in these patients, covered SEMS are considered the treatment of choice in patients with malignant esophago-respiratory fistula.

References

1. Shin JH, Song HY, Ko GY, et al. Esophagorespiratory fistula: long-term results of palliative treatment with covered expandable metallic stents in 61 patients. *Radiology.* 2004;232(1):252-259.
2. Sharma P, Kozarek R, and the Practice Parameters Committee of the American College of Gastroenterology. Role of esophageal stents in benign and malignant diseases. *Am J Gastroenterol.* 2010;105(2):258-273.

A 55-Year-Old Man Undergoes an Esophagectomy for Esophageal Cancer. Two Years Later, He Develops Dysphagia and a Contrast Study Discloses a Narrowing at His Anastomosis. How Should This Be Investigated and Treated?

Michael Walker, MD and John Fang, MD

In the above case, radiologic evaluation has identified a stricture at the anastomosis from the previous esophagectomy. The main differential for this finding is a benign anastomotic stricture versus a recurrent malignant stricture. Dysphagia due to anatomical narrowing usually requires approximately 50% occlusion of the esophageal lumen. Patients in this situation will initially have solid food dysphagia, with dysphagia for liquids indicating more severe narrowing. Other important signs and symptoms to inquire about include weight loss, chest pain, reflux, and aspiration. Most patients in this setting can now proceed to upper endoscopy. Endoscopic appearance of the anastomotic stricture usually suggests whether a stricture is benign or malignant, but biopsies should be obtained if there is any concern about recurrent malignancy.

Benign Stricture

Benign esophageal strictures are classified as simple or complex. Simple strictures are straight and short (< 1 cm) and can be easily passed with a normal diameter (8 to 10 mm) endoscope. These include peptic strictures, Schatzki's rings, and esophageal webs. Complex strictures are often longer (> 2 cm), angulated, and sufficiently narrow that

Figure 6-1. Endoscopic image of a benign anastomotic stricture following esopha-gectomy. The stenosis was 15-mm long and 5-mm wide.

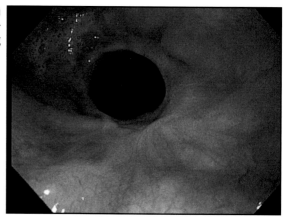

passing a normal diameter endoscope is difficult. Complex strictures are due to radiation, photodynamic therapy, caustic ingestions, and surgical anastomoses. Complex strictures are often refractory to treatment. Refractory strictures are defined as those that cannot be dilated to 14 mm over 5 sessions at 2-week intervals. Recurrent strictures are defined as those that do not maintain satisfactory luminal diameter for 4 weeks after dilation to at least 14 mm.[1] This patient most likely has a benign anastomotic stricture and thus is more likely to be refractory and recurrent.

Anastomotic strictures have been noted to occur in up to 30% to 42% of patients who undergo esophagectomy. Pre-existing cardiac disease, diabetes mellitus, postoperative anastomotic leaks, ischemia of the gastric conduit, and stapled (versus hand-sewn) anas-tomosis all increase the likelihood of developing an anastomotic stricture (Figure 6-1).

Treatment of Benign Anastomotic Strictures

Dilation remains the first-line therapy for benign strictures. Balloon dilation (radial force alone) compared to bougie dilation (radial and shear force) shows no difference in treatment outcomes.[2]

Several studies have validated the use of dilation in treating benign anastomotic post-esophagectomy strictures. A mean of 3 to 5 sessions is generally required, regardless of whether balloons or bougies were used.[3-5]

Intralesional steroid injections have been shown to increase time between dila-tions, increase end dilation diameter size, and decrease the total number of dilations.[6,7] Additional adjuvant therapy can be considered if dilation and intralesional steroids do not improve or maintain improvement of dysphagia. Needle-knife electrocautery (to incise the stricture itself) for the treatment of benign anastomotic strictures (BAS) has been described in patients refractory to dilation.[8] A study of 62 patients with BAS randomized to treatment with Savary dilation or electrocautery incision found no difference in success rate between the 2 treatment groups.[9]

Another modality for management of complex anastomotic stricture is the placement of an esophageal stent (Figure 6-2). Both self-expanding metal stents (SEMS) and self-expanding plastic stents (SEPS) have been used in this setting. Initial reports of SEPS use in BAS were encouraging with 95% to 100% placement success rates and overall success

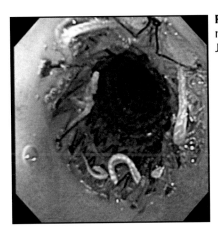

Figure 6-2. Same patient as Figure 6-1, following placement of an Alimaxx-E (Merit Medical Systems, Inc, South Jordan, UT) fully covered self-expanding metal stent.

of up to 80%.[10] However, more recent reports have demonstrated migration rates as high as 75% with up to 90% of patients developing recurrent strictures after stent removal.[11,12] SEMS are available in partially covered and fully covered versions. In a review of 29 patients receiving partially covered SEMS for benign strictures, 80% had major complications, including stent migration (31%), chest pain or reflux (21%), tracheoesophageal fistula (6%), anemia (3%), and new stricture formation (41%).[13] Fully covered metal stents are potentially removable after placement and are useful in refractory anastomotic stricture.

Finally, patients having continued symptomatic strictures can be considered for self-bougienage using Maloney dilators. Patients are given a Maloney dilator both less than 50 French and smaller than the greatest size achieved with endoscopic dilation. Patients should also be considered for surgical revision with colonic interposition, although this carries significant morbidity and can be technically challenging.

Evaluation and Management of Malignant Stricture

Malignant strictures due to recurrent cancer portend a poor prognosis. Recurrent esophageal cancer occurs locally 30% to 40% of the time and is best diagnosed with endoscopy and biopsy. Treatment modalities including radiation therapy, chemotherapy, repeat surgical intervention, or palliative therapy should be discussed in a multidisciplinary team including the gastroenterologist, medical oncologist, surgeon, and radiation oncologist. The role of the gastroenterologist in the treatment of a recurrent malignant esophageal stricture focuses on palliation of symptoms of dysphagia, generally via endoscopic stent placement.

Uncovered, partially covered, and fully covered SEMS as well as SEPS have all been reported to be successful in the palliation of malignant esophageal strictures. The overall success rate is 70% to 90% with a complication rate of 30% to 35%.[14,15] Major complications include hemorrhage, perforation, fistula, and fever, while minor complications include chest pain, tissue ingrowth or overgrowth, food impaction, and stent migration.[15] These are all less commonly encountered when the stents are placed via experienced operators. Partially covered esophageal stents have the best balance between preventing ingrowth and reducing migration rates and are presently the stent of choice in palliating unresectable malignant esophageal strictures.

Clinical Practice

We suspect that the patient has a benign anastomotic stricture and, less likely, a recurrent malignant stricture. We would first proceed to upper endoscopy with biopsy. At this initial endoscopy, we would perform dilation for immediate symptom improvement, regardless of malignant or benign etiology. If the lesion is malignant, referral to a multidisciplinary oncology team for additional re-staging is warranted. If palliation of symptoms is desired, we would proceed with partially covered SEMS placement.

If the biopsy is negative for malignancy and our suspicion is confirmed that this is a benign anastomotic stricture, we follow the patient symptomatically. If symptoms recur, we continue with repeat dilations every 2 to 4 weeks and initiate adjuvant steroid injections at all subsequent endoscopies. If after 3 to 5 dilations with adjuvant steroids the patient has a refractory/recurrent stricture, we would consider the use of electrocautery incision and/or stent placement versus continued dilation depending on the frequency and maximal diameter of dilation. Our overall treatment protocol for management of esophageal strictures is shown in Figure 6-3.

References

1. Kochman M, McClave S, Boyce H. The refractory and recurrent esophageal stricture: a definition. *Gastrointest Endosc.* 2005;62(3):474-475.
2. Scolapio J, Pasha T, Gostout C, et al. A randomized prospective study comparing rigid to balloon dilators for benign esophageal strictures and rings. *Gastrointest Endosc.* 1999;50(1):13-17.
3. Honkoop P, Siersma P, Tilanus H, Stassen L, Hop W, van Blankenstein M. Benign anastomotic strictures after transhiatal esophagectomy and cervical esophagogastrostomy: risk factor and management. *J Thorac Cardiovasc Surg.* 1996;111(6):1141-1146.
4. Pereira-Lima J, Ramires R, Zamin I Jr, Cassal A, Marroni C, Mattos A. Endoscopic dilation of benign esophageal strictures; report on 1043 procedures. *Am J Gastroenterol.* 1999;94(6):1497-1501.
5. Williams V, Watson T, Zhovtis S, et al. Endoscopic and symptomatic assessment of anastomotic strictures following esophagectomy and cervical esophagogastrostomy. *Surg Endosc.* 2008;22(6):1470-1476.
6. Ramage J Jr, Rumalla A, Baron T, et al. A prospective, randomized, double-blind, placebo-controlled trial of endoscopic steroid injection therapy for recalcitrant esophageal peptic strictures. *Am J Gastroenterol.* 2005;100(11):2419-2425.
7. Altintas E, Kacar S, Tunc B, et al. Usefulness of intralesional triamcinolone in treatment of benign esophageal strictures. *Gastrointest Endosc.* 2002;56(6):829-834.
8. Hordijk M, Siersma P, Tilanus H, Kuipers E. Electrocautery therapy for refractory anastomotic strictures of the esophagus. *Gastrointest Endosc.* 2006;63(1):157-163.
9. Hordijk M, van Hooft J, Hansen B, Fockens P, Kuipers E. A randomized comparison of electrocautery incision with Savary bougienage for relief of anastomotic gastroesophageal strictures. *Gastrointest Endosc.* 2009;70(5):849-855.
10. Evrad S, Le Moine O, Lazaraki G, Dormann A, El Nakadi I, Deviere J. Self-expanding plastic stents for benign esophageal lesions. *Gastrointest Endosc.* 2004;60(6):894-900.
11. Dua K, Vieggaar F, Santharam R, Siersema P. Removable self-expanding plastic esophageal stent as a continuous, non-permanent dilator in treating refractory benign esophageal strictures: a prospective two-center study. *Am J Gastroenterol.* 2008;103(12):2988-2994.
12. Holm A, de la Mora Levy J, Gostout C, Topazian M, Baron T. Self-expanding plastic stents in the treatment of benign esophageal conditions. *Gastrointest Endosc.* 2008;67(1):20-25.
13. Sandha GS, Marcon NE. Expandable metal stents for benign esophageal obstruction. *Gastrointest Endosc Clin N Am.* 1999;9(3):437-446.
14. Siersema PD, de Wijkerslooth LR. Dilation of refractory benign esophageal strictures. *Gastrointest Endosc.* 2009;70(5):1000-1012.
15. Sharma P, Kozarek R. Practice Parameters of the American College of Gastroenterology. Role of esophageal stents in benign and malignant disease. *Am J Gastroenterol.* 2010;105(2):258-273.

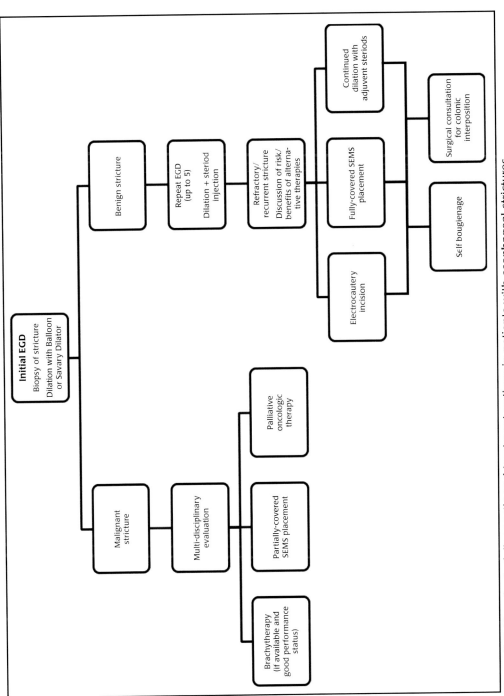

Figure 6-3. Flowchart of diagnostic and treatment options in patients with esophageal strictures.

SECTION II

GASTRIC

QUESTION

WHAT ARE THE KNOWN RISK FACTORS FOR THE DEVELOPMENT OF GASTRIC CANCER?

Selvi Thirumurthi, MD, MS

Gastric cancer (adenocarcinoma) is recognized as the fourth most common cancer and carries a high mortality rate. Gastric cancer presents a significant public health challenge, especially among developing countries where incidence rates are highest. There are several known risk factors for gastric cancer, but it is important to first distinguish the 2 types of gastric cancer. The intestinal type manifests as a gastric mass and is more closely associated with environmental risk factors that will be discussed below. The diffuse type is poorly differentiated and carries a worse prognosis than the intestinal type.

The most widely recognized risk factor for gastric cancer is *Helicobacter pylori* infection. *H. pylori* has been identified by the World Health Organization as a class I carcinogen for gastric cancer and gastric lymphoma. *H. pylori* were first cultured in 1983 by Warren and Marshall, and subsequent investigators have demonstrated the link between *H. pylori*, gastritis, and gastric adenocarcinoma.[1] Why does *H. pylori* (or any other) gastritis increase the risk of cancer? Chronic gastritis can evolve into gastric atrophy if the inciting agent is not removed. Ongoing inflammation results in continuing damage to the mucosa, leading to atrophy and the development of a metaplastic epithelium, either pyloric or mucous metaplasia, or intestinal metaplasia. These metaplastic epithelia are the fertile soil in which cancer can develop. Some strains of *H. pylori* infection, such as those with the CagA pathogenicity island, are more virulent in that they cause increased degrees of inflammation and thus have greater carcinogenic potential. This sequence of events has been described as the Correa pathway (Figure 7-1).[2]

What is the pathophysiology behind the progression of these precursor lesions to gastric cancer? In atrophic gastritis, loss of parietal cell mass results in diminished acid production. This creates an environment that may encourage colonization with bacteria that are capable of converting dietary nitrates to nitrites that can eventually become mutagenic N-nitroso compounds. Because normal gastric acid levels are required to maintain

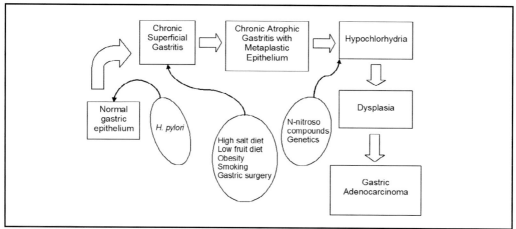

Figure 7-1. Correa pathway, highlighting the sequence of events leading to gastric cancer.

normal levels of serum gastrin, an excess of gastrin can occur in patients with atrophic gastritis. Gastrin has a potent proliferative effect on gastric mucosa and thus may play a role in tumor growth.[3]

There are several ways to test your patient for *H. pylori* infection. Tests include a simple blood test to detect antibodies against *H. pylori*, endoscopic biopsies, stool antigen tests, and breath tests to check for the presence of urease produced by *H. pylori*. Once you have diagnosed your patient with *H. pylori*, it is important to treat the infection and then confirm eradication. This can be accomplished by the stool or breath tests or mucosal biopsies if repeat endoscopy is planned.

There are also dietary risk factors for gastric cancer. The accumulation of N-nitroso compounds has been linked to the development of gastric cancer. These compounds, which are widely employed, are found in certain fertilizers and in pickled or smoked foods. A diet low in fruits and vegetables has also been linked to gastric cancer. Adequate levels of vitamin C act to reduce the formation of N-nitroso compounds. High salt intake has been linked to the formation of chronic gastritis and may be particularly harmful in patients with *H. pylori* infection and/or atrophic gastritis.

Obesity is a significant public health concern and has also been linked to the development of gastric cancer. The risk of gastric cancer was shown to increase with increasing body mass index (BMI) in a recent study with an overall relative risk of 1.22 for patients with BMI greater than 25. This effect was significant among non-Asians compared to Asian patients (OR 1.24).[4]

Smoking has also been linked to gastric cancer. A recent meta-analysis evaluated the relationship between smoking and gastric cancer. The relative risk of developing gastric cancer was 1.7 among heavy smokers (more than 30 cigarettes a day) and 1.3 for lighter smokers. Former smokers had an intermediate risk for gastric cancer compared to those who had never smoked.[5]

Not only do environmental risk factors play a role in gastric cancer, but genetic predispositions also play a role. Individuals with a first-degree family member with gastric cancer are at a 2- to 3-fold risk of developing it as well, likely due to similar genetic make-up and environmental exposures. Those with a family history of familial adenomatous polyposis (FAP) or hereditary nonpolyposis syndrome (HNPCC) are also at increased risk for gastric cancer.

Overall, the known risk factors for gastric cancer include genetic predispositions and environmental exposures. The best recognized environmental risk factor is *H. pylori* infection, which also clusters in families. It is important to identify patients with *H. pylori* infection in order to treat and eradicate this carcinogenic pathogen, which should impact the incidence of gastric cancer. It is also imperative to remember the other risk factors in order to diagnose gastric cancer at the earliest possible stage to improve patient outcomes.

References

1. Marshall BJ, Warren JR. Unidentified curved bacilli in the stomach of patients with gastritis and peptic ulceration. *Lancet.* 1984;323(8390):1311-1315.
2. Houghton JM, Wang T. Tumors of the stomach. In: Feldman M, Friedman L, eds. *Sleisenger & Fordtran's Gastrointestinal and Liver Disease.* Philadelphia, PA: Saunders Elsevier Incorporated; 2006:1139-1157.
3. Graham DY, Asaka M. Eradication of gastric cancer and more efficient gastric cancer surveillance in Japan: two peas in a pod. *J Gastroenterol.* 2010;45(1):1-8.
4. Yang P, Zhou Y, Chen B, et al. Overweight, obesity and gastric cancer risk: results from a meta-analysis of cohort studies. *Eur J Cancer.* 2009;45(16):2867-2873.
5. Ladeiras-Lopes R, Pereira K, Nogueira A, et al. Smoking and gastric cancer: systematic review and meta-analysis of cohort studies. *Cancer Causes Control.* 2008;19(7):689-701.

What Is the Relationship Between Helicobacter pylori and the Development of Gastric Cancer and Lymphoma? Do All Patients With Helicobacter pylori-Related Gastric Malignancies Need Surgery?

Scott Pollack, MD and Virendra Joshi, MD, AGAF

Helicobacter pylori infection is found in approximately half of the world's population and has been shown to be involved in several gastroduodenal diseases, namely peptic ulcer disease, gastric cancer, and mucosa-associated lymphoid tissue (MALT) lymphoma. Most individuals who are infected with *H. pylori* remain asymptomatic throughout life. *H. pylori* has been deemed a class I carcinogen by the World Health Organization (WHO), and there are several mechanisms by which this gram-negative bacterium has been implicated in the pathologic changes leading to dysplasia and malignancy.

Gastric cancer is currently the fourth most common cancer in the world and the second most common cause of cancer-related mortality. Nonetheless, its incidence is quite low in North America.[1] In Japan, where the incidence of gastric cancer is relatively high, there are screening programs in place to diagnose gastric cancer in its earlier or precursor stages, thus improving mortality rates. In the United States, the diagnosis is most commonly made in the later stages of the disease, resulting in a higher mortality. The most common sites for gastric adenocarcinoma diagnosis in North America are not within the distal stomach, as is seen in developing countries, but in the proximal stomach along the lesser

Figure 8-1. Ulcerated mass on the lesser curvature at endoscopy. Biopsy revealed gastric adenocarcinoma.

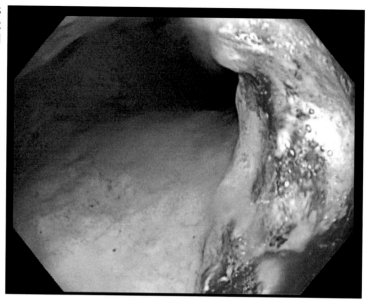

curvature, in the cardia, and at the level of the gastroesophageal junction (Figure 8-1). This fact is likely explained by the aggressive detection and treatment of *H. pylori* infection in recent years.

It is well known that both bacterial and host factors play a role in the pathogenesis of *H. pylori*-associated malignancies. The direct effects of mucosal infection by *H. pylori* lead to multiple histological changes. There are changes seen within the gastric epithelial lining including an increased presence of leukocytes as well as multiple oxidative stresses caused directly by infection of this bacterium. Oxidative stress can be caused by the production of superoxides by the bacteria itself, increased production of reactive oxygen species by the epithelium as a result of infection, and reduced levels of the antioxidant vitamin C, all leading to increased inflammation and cell turnover.

Host factors, such as dietary and lifestyle factors, may play a role in gastric cancer pathogenesis beyond the role of *H. pylori*. These include a high salt intake and a lack of antioxidants from fruits and vegetables, and there is a proposed role of dietary N-nitroso compounds in the intestinal metaplasia to carcinoma sequence.

Genetic mutations of the tumor suppressor genes p53 and adenomatous polyposis coli (APC), a loss of deleted in colon cancer (DCC), macrosatellite instability, and germline mutations of the E-cadherin/CDH1 gene have been implicated as well. *H. pylori* can also disrupt the homeostasis of the gastric mucosa by causing epithelial proliferation, inducing apoptosis, and activating tyrosine kinase receptors. This can then lead to atrophy, inflammation, achlorhydria, bacterial overgrowth, and increased cell turnover, all of which predispose the patient to the development of dysplasia. Several bacterial virulence factors have been widely studied and theorized to be involved in the pathogenesis of malignancy. One such factor is CagA, a protein involved in the secretion system of the bacterium, which has been shown to interact with the signal-transduction pathways present in gastric epithelial cells. Studies have shown that those with certain CagA strains have a higher relative risk for gastric cancer.[2]

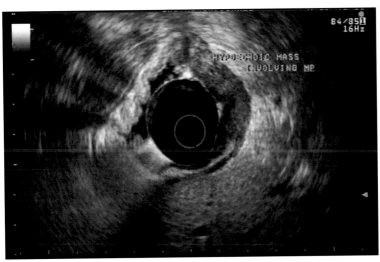

Figure 8-2. Endoscopic ultrasound image of the mass seen in Figure 8-1. The mass was found to be penetrating the muscularis propria of gastric wall, but without associated adenopathy, consistent with locoregional tumor stage T3N0.

The preceding factors are theorized to be the main culprits in the pathogenesis of *H. pylori* infection-related malignancy. The progression is seen as a series of events starting from normal mucosa and leading to superficial gastritis, atrophic gastritis, intestinal metaplasia, dysplasia, and eventually cancer.[3] It has been shown that the eradication of *H. pylori* infection can lead to the improvement of gastritis and inflammation, yet there is conflicting evidence that treatment will reverse changes consistent with more advanced changes, such as atrophic gastritis or metaplasia. Randomized trials have shown both regression and nonregression of intestinal metaplasia after treatment for *H. pylori*, and more long-term studies are necessary to resolve this issue.

A key clinical issue is the utility of endoscopic surveillance of those with intestinal metaplasia of the stomach. Several population studies have shown that surveillance can diagnose gastric cancer in its earlier stages. At our center, we choose to perform surveillance of these patients every 1 to 3 years by standard endoscopy and also to perform advanced imaging techniques, such as probe- or endoscope-based confocal laser endomicroscopy using fluorescein dye.

MALT lymphomas of the stomach are frequently associated with concurrent *H. pylori* infection. The pathogenesis of these lesions is explained by the proliferation of neoplastic B cells stimulated by T-cell activation of antigen presenting cells carrying *H. pylori* proteins. A high percentage of these lymphomas respond to standard therapy for *H. pylori* and have a favorable outcome.

The treatments for gastric adenocarcinoma and MALT lymphoma differ greatly, despite their often sharing the characteristic of concurrent infection with *H. pylori*. Surgery is the main treatment for gastric adenocarcinoma along with eradication of *H. pylori* if the patient is symptomatic. For most MALT lymphomas, especially in the early stage, the primary treatment is eradication of *H. pylori*.

The initial work-up after a diagnosis of gastric adenocarcinoma is to obtain baseline laboratory blood work and imaging studies to stage the cancer. Accurate staging of the cancer will direct further treatment. Initial staging is often obtained with computed topography (CT) of the abdomen. An endoscopic ultrasound (EUS) may be done for more accurate staging when available (Figure 8-2). The role of EUS is well established in assessing the involvement of adenocarcinoma within the gastric wall layers and is superior to other imaging modalities. High-frequency miniprobes using 20-MHz frequency are suggested to give better wall layer delineation (resolution) than standard 7- to 12-MHz echoendoscopes, suggesting the efficacy of high-frequency probes in detecting early gastric cancer. The accuracy of establishing nodal stage by EUS, however, is low, as perigastric or gastrohepatic nodes can be difficult to fully detect. EUS has an additional diagnostic advantage in that it can also be used to sample small amounts of ascitic fluid for cytology.

At the time of endoscopy in patients with gastric adenocarcinoma, *H. pylori* testing should be performed. If present, and if the patient is symptomatic, it is eradicated with standard treatment consisting of a triple regimen of double-dose proton pump inhibitor, clarithromycin, and amoxicillin/metronidazole. If a cancerous lesion is found early and only involves the mucosa without invading the submucosa, the patient can be given the option to undergo endoscopic mucosal resection (EMR), especially if he or she has significant comorbidities or a poor performance status, or he or she can undergo a gastrectomy. For more invasive disease, surgery is combined with neoadjuvant and adjuvant chemotherapy. Alternatively, patients may also be given radiation after surgery, especially if positive surgical margins are present. In patients with metastatic disease or if the patient is medically unfit for surgery, palliative chemotherapy is typically offered.[4] Early gastric cancer detection and resection by EMR is not very common in the United States because, unlike in Japan, aggressive gastric cancer surveillance strategies are not prevalent and most cancers are already in an advanced stage at the time of diagnosis.

For MALT lymphomas, the initial diagnostic work-up includes a thorough review of the initial pathology specimens for distinct histological changes and immunophenotyping in order to verify the diagnosis. Often, further investigation in the form of molecular genetic analysis and cytogenetics is performed looking for unfavorable genetic arrangements. *H. pylori* infection is determined by histologic evaluation, fluorescent in situ hybridization, or other noninvasive testing. CT scans, positron emission tomography (PET), and EUS are useful to determine the depth of invasion of the gastric wall, lymph nodes status, and distant metastases.

If the patient is found to be *H. pylori* positive and the lesion is localized to the gastric wall, then the initial treatment is standard therapy for the bacterial infection with verification of eradication with repeat endoscopy 3 months later. Even if the lesion penetrates the gastric serosa and involves adjacent organs but no lymph nodes are involved, the initial therapy is a non-surgical approach, assuming the patient is *H. pylori* positive. Those who do not respond are usually patients with a more advanced stage or who have a distinct genetic profile, t(11;18) (q21;q21) translocation. These can be irradiated successfully if the tumors have only locoregional spread. If there is systemic involvement, then these patients are generally candidates for a monoclonal antibody against B-cells (rituximab) with or without chemotherapy. Once patients are treated successfully, they need to be followed long-term for possible relapse.

If the patient is *H. pylori* negative by multiple testing modalities, then he or she is offered radiation therapy or rituximab with or without chemotherapy.[4] Treatment guidelines are summarized in Table 8-1. No firm guidelines exist for the endoscopic surveillance of those who have been successfully treated. At our center, we perform surveillance endoscopic exams every 1 to 5 years, based on symptomatology and clinical situation, after index endoscopy confirming the histologic remission of MALT.

<u>Table 8-1</u>

Treatment Schema for Gastric Cancer by Stage

Treatment for Gastric Adenocarcinoma by Stage		
AJCC Staging	*Tumor Description*	*Treatment*
0	Carcinoma in situ	EMR/ESD or Surgery
IA	Invades lamina propria (T1a), muscularis mucosa (T1a), or submucosa (T1b)	
IB	Invades muscularis propria and/or submucosa with/without 1 to 2 lymph nodes	Surgery/adj. therapy
IIA	Invades subserosal connective tissue or invades less deeply with lymph node involvement	Surgery/adj. therapy
IIB	Invades serosa or invades less deeply with lymph node involvement	Surgery/adj. therapy
IIIA	Invades serosa with lymph node involvement or invades less deeply with greater lymph node involvement	Surgery/adj. therapy
IIIB	Invades adjacent structures with/without lymph node involvement or invades less deeply with a greater lymph node involvement.	Surgery/adj. therapy
IIIC	Invades adjacent structures with greater lymph node involvement	Surgery/adj. therapy
IV	Distant Metastasis	Palliation

Treatment for MALT Lymphoma by Stage				
Lugano Staging	*TNM Staging*	*Description*		*Treatment*
I	T1 N0 M0	Confined to the GI Tract	Tumor extends to mucosa/submucosa	If *H. pylori* positive, then treat with standard therapy, otherwise RT or rituximab
	T2 N0 M0		Tumor extends to muscularis propria	
	T3 N0 M0		Tumor extends to serosa	
II	T1-3 N1 M0	Tumor extends into the abdomen	Perigastric lymph nodes involved	
	T1-3 N2 M0		Distant regional lymph nodes involved	
II$_E$	T4 N0 M0	Tumor penetrates serosa and involves adjacent organs/structures		
III-IV	T1-4 N3 M0	Disseminated lymph node involvement and/or involvement of lymph nodes on both sides of the diaphragm		Chemo-immunotherapy or RT
	T1-4 N0-3 M1			

AJCC indicates American Joint Committee on Cancer; EMR, endoscopic mucosal resection; ESD, endoscopic submucosal dissection (both should be performed at an experienced center); TNM, tumor, node, metastasis; RT, radiation therapy; adj, adjuvant.

References

1. Kamanger F, Dores GM, Anderson WF. Patterns of cancer incidence, mortality, and prevalence across five continents: defining priorities to reduce cancer disparities in different geographic regions of the world. *J Clin Oncol.* 2006;24(14):2137-2150.

2. Huang JQ, Zheng GF, Sumanac K, Irvine EJ, Hunt RH. Meta-analysis of the relationship between CagA seropositivity and gastric cancer. *Gastroenterology.* 2003;125(6):1636-1644.

3. Correa P. Human gastric carcinogenesis: a multistep and multifactorial process—First American Cancer Society Award Lecture on Cancer Epidemiology and Prevention. *Cancer Res.* 1992;52(24):6735-6740.

4. National Comprehensive Cancer Network. NCCN clinical practice guidelines in oncology: gastric cancer and non-Hodgkin's lymphoma. http://www.nccn.org/professionals/physician_gls/f_guidelines.asp. 2010. Accessed March 10, 2010.

WHAT OPTIONS EXIST FOR PATIENTS WITH GASTRIC OUTLET OBSTRUCTION FROM GASTRIC CANCER?

Andrew Singleton, MD and Robert E. Glasgow, MD

The patient with obstructing gastric cancer can be a difficult challenge for the practicing gastroenterologist. This chapter will review the medical, endoscopic, and surgical options for relieving obstruction.

Differential Diagnosis of Malignant Obstruction

The differential diagnosis for malignant gastric outlet obstruction includes primary gastric malignancies (adenocarcinoma, lymphomas, gastrointestinal stromal tumors, and carcinoid) and perigastric or periampullary malignancies (pancreatic, duodenal, or ampullary adenocarcinoma, cholangiocarcinoma, extragastric lymphomas, and perigastric metastases) as well as several benign conditions. For the purposes of this discussion, we will focus on gastric outlet obstruction from gastric adenocarcinoma.

Gastric cancer is still the world's second leading cause of cancer mortality, second only to lung cancer, although 15% to 20% of pancreatic cancer patients will develop gastric outlet obstruction during the course of their treatment.[1,2] Endoscopic biopsy and complete radiographic characterization by computed tomography scan is vital in identifying the cause of obstruction and, in the case of malignant obstruction, in providing for adequate staging of the underlying cancer.

No matter the cause, clinical presentation usually involves vomiting, nausea, malnutrition, dehydration, and associated electrolyte abnormalities. Malignant gastric outlet obstruction can go unrecognized until severe malnutrition has already been established. This is often seen in patients receiving chemoradiation in whom nausea and vomiting are attributed to these therapies instead of the actual underlying mechanical obstruction.

Two important items in a patient's clinical history that should trigger your suspicion for malignant obstruction are vomiting undigested food and nonbilious emesis.

Surgical Options

Surgical options for the patient with gastric outlet obstruction include both resection and bypass. All patients with resectable disease whose overall health would permit a major operation should undergo resection. Management of these patients should be reviewed in a multidisciplinary fashion in concert with the medical and radiation oncologists, as most patients will require either neoadjuvant treatment or adjuvant chemoradiotherapy. Resection with a distal or total gastrectomy depends upon tumor size and location. Distal lesions are amenable to subtotal gastrectomy with either Billroth II gastrojejunostomy or Roux-en-Y reconstruction. For distal gastrectomy, a 5-cm margin of grossly normal stomach is required to ensure negative microscopic margins. Total gastrectomy with Roux-en-Y esophagojejunostomy is required for bulky tumors that involve the body and fundus of the stomach. In patients with metastatic disease and gastric outlet obstruction, a palliative distal gastrectomy can be performed if technically feasible, if patient comorbidities are favorable, and if a limited extent of metastatic disease is present. A total gastrectomy for palliation should be discouraged because of excessive morbidity.

If not resectable, the goal of palliative surgery in the obstructed patient with gastric cancer is maximal relief of obstructive symptoms with minimal morbidity. Options include endoscopic, percutaneous, or surgical tube gastrostomy for decompression and surgical jejunostomy for enteral access. Open and laparoscopic gastrojejunostomy bypass is technically simple and can be done with low morbidity (Figure 9-1). Occasionally, surgical, radiographic, or endoscopic treatment of concomitant biliary obstruction is necessary. These modalities are best applied to patients with a greater than 6-month anticipated survival and no peritoneal disease, hepatic metastasis, ascites, diffuse nodal metastases, or proximal gastric outlet obstruction. The laparoscopic approach is now commonplace with decreased blood loss, decreased time to solid food intake, and decreased complications but no difference in length of stay when compared to open gastrojejunostomy.[3] Complications related to gastrojejunostomy include bleeding, infection, damage to associated structures, and the more procedure-specific risks of anastomotic leak, efferent or afferent loop obstruction, marginal ulcer, and anastomotic stricture.[3]

Endoscopic Options

Nonsurgical options for management of gastric outlet obstruction from gastric cancer include balloon dilation, percutaneous endoscopic gastrostomy tubes with jejunal extensions for feeding, and enteral stenting (ES). Balloon dilation is technically simple and inexpensive but has uniformly short-lived efficacy. Dilation may serve to facilitate other more lasting options. Gastrostomy tubes may be placed endoscopically or via interventional radiology.

Palliative stenting of the gastroduodenal region has gained widespread acceptance. Stenting has the advantage of preserving normal oral nutrition. The stents currently used are metal expandable mesh (Figure 9-2). The goal of endoscopic stenting is to restore and maintain patency, re-establishing continuity between the stomach and duodenum. The

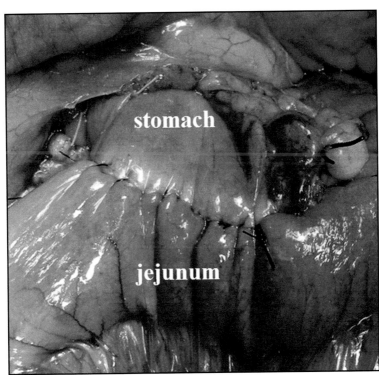

Figure 9-1. Intraoperative photo of a newly created surgical gastro-jejunostomy showing the anastomosis between the small bowel and the stomach.

stents pass through the operating channel of a therapeutic endoscope and are used with fluoroscopic guidance for precise localization of obstruction and dimensional information about the obstruction, which is crucial to stent length selection and placement.

Reported clinical success rates of endoscopic stenting range from 79% to 91% depending on the outcome measures used. The most common of these are improvement in obstructive symptoms (nausea/vomiting), resumption of a solid or soft diet, or change in the gastric outlet obstruction scoring system score developed by Adler and Baron.[4] Complications of ES have been categorized as immediate, early, or late. Immediate complications occur within 24 hours and include bleeding and perforation. Early complications occur up to 2 to 4 weeks after stent placement. Early complications include stent positioning problems, perforation, bleeding, and aspiration. Late complications include reobstruction, stent migration, bleeding, and a single reported case of aortoenteric fistula from stent erosion. Uncovered metal stents have been compared to covered stents with results showing an increased incidence of tumor overgrowth into uncovered stents and a stent migration rate of 21% to 26% in covered stents, requiring an increased rate of re-intervention.[5] In our patient, the presence of what appears to be profound gastric tumor involvement may reduce the chances of a good clinical outcome as there is likely to be little to no gastric motility even after stenting, and the patient may only be able to take liquids.

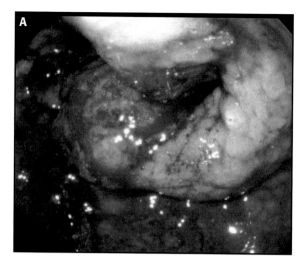

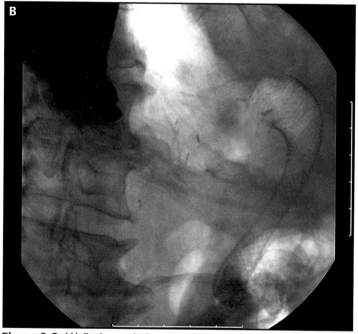

Figure 9-2. (A) Endoscopic image of the pylorus in a patient with malignant gastric outlet obstruction due to gastric cancer. The distal stomach has been completely infiltrated with malignant tissue, the pylorus is stenosed, and there is no functional peristalsis in the stomach. (Reprinted wtih permission from Douglas G. Adler, MD, FACG, AGAF, FASGE.) (B) Fluoroscopic image of the same patient following placement of a stent across the pylorus into the pylorus and proximal duodenum. (Reprinted with permission of Douglas G. Adler, MD.)

Endoscopy Versus Surgery

A recent comprehensive review of 13 studies comparing surgical and endoscopic modalities was published, including a total of 514 patients. Patients undergoing ES were more likely to ever tolerate an oral diet (soft or solid), have a shorter mean time to oral intake (7 days), and have a shorter length of stay. Of note, there were no differences in survival or 30-day mortality between the ES and surgical groups. Open gastrojejunostomy patients were found to have more "major" complications, including respiratory tract infections, myocardial infarction, acute renal failure, and wound infection, but better long-term patency. Only 3 studies in this review looked at laparoscopic gastrojejunostomy (LGJ) compared to ES. Average length of stay was shorter for the ES group. LGJ patients had more complications and longer mean time to tolerate a diet. Average patient survival was improved in the LGJ group compared to the ES patients.[6] Most studies conclude that long-term patency is superior with bypass over stenting with fewer secondary interventions to maintain patency, supporting the recommendation that patients with a longer life expectancy be considered for surgical gastrojejunostomy.[2]

Radiation and Chemotherapy

Radiation therapy has been shown to improve symptoms associated with gastric cancer, including dysphagia/obstruction, bleeding, and pain in patients not fit for other palliative modalities. In a recent review, 81% (13 of 16) of patients were shown to have obstructive/dysphagia symptoms controlled by radiation therapy for a median time of 81% of remaining life.[7] While effective in palliating malignant obstruction, radiotherapy will take at least 2 to 3 weeks to achieve peak benefits, which may be too long for some patients facing profound failure to thrive.

The addition of chemotherapy to ES for gastric outlet obstruction from gastric cancer has been shown to improve long-term patency. Chemotherapy, along with radiation therapy, is commonly prescribed to gastric cancer patients in either a neoadjuvant setting, adjuvant setting, or for palliation of bleeding and gastric outlet obstruction. According to the National Comprehensive Cancer Network guidelines, response rates to these therapies may range from 10% to 20%, and a variety of agents are available.[8]

References

1. Kelley JR, Duggan JM. Gastric cancer epidemiology and risk factors. *J Clin Epidemiol.* 2003;56(1):1-9.
2. Jeurnink SM, van Eijck CH, Steyerberg EW, et al. Stent versus gastrojejunostomy for the palliation of gastric outlet obstruction: a systematic review. *BMC Gastroenterol.* 2007;7:18.
3. Navarra G, Musolino C, Venneri A, et al. Palliative antecolic isoperistaltic gastrojejunostomy: a randomized controlled trial comparing open and laparoscopic approaches. *Surg Endosc.* 2006;20(12):1831-1834.
4. Adler DG, Baron TH. Endoscopic palliation of malignant gastric outlet obstruction using self-expanding metal stents: experience in 36 patients. *Am J Gastroenterol.* 2002;97(1):72-78.
5. Gaidos JK, Draganov PV. Treatment of malignant gastric outlet obstruction with endoscopically placed self-expandable metal stents. *World J Gastroenterol.* 2009;15(35):4365-4371.
6. Jasen L, Gregory O, Mittai A, et al. A systematic review of methods to palliate malignant gastric outlet obstruction. *Surg Endosc.* 2010;24(2):290-297.
7. Kim MM, Rana V, Janjan NA, et al. Clinical benefit of palliative radiation therapy in advanced gastric cancer. *Acta Oncol.* 2008;47(3):421-427.
8. Ajani JA, Barthel JS, Bekaii-Saab T, et al. Gastric cancer. *J Natl Compr Canc Netw.* 2010;8(4):378-409.

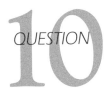
WHAT IS THE ROLE OF ENDOSCOPIC ULTRASOUND IN STAGING GASTRIC CANCERS?

Jeffrey L. Tokar, MD

Endoscopic ultrasound (EUS) for the evaluation of gastric lesions is a common indication for referral to my endoscopy unit. EUS, with or without fine needle aspiration (FNA), plays an important and sometimes pivotal role in the evaluation of gastric pathology. EUS can help differentiate neoplastic from non-neoplastic endoscopic findings and may be useful in the pretreatment staging of gastric malignancies, specifically gastric adenocarcinoma.

Basic Principles of Gastric Endoscopic Ultrasound

Radial echoendoscopes provide a 360-degree view, resolve the gastric wall in a 5-echolayer pattern (Figure 10-1A), and visualize structures within and adjacent to the stomach. High-frequency ultrasound miniprobes (HFUMP) allow greater resolution of the gastric wall layers into 7 to 9 echolayers (Figure 10-1B), but provide limited information about structures outside the gastric wall (eg, lymph nodes, liver). Curvilinear array echoendoscopes enable FNA but do not provide a 360-degree view, and the 5-layer wall pattern is often harder to appreciate with these devices than with radial echoendoscopes. In general, I use HFUMPs to evaluate smaller localized lesions, such as early stage gastric cancers, to assess candidacy for endoscopic resection (Figure 10-2). Radial/curvilinear echoendoscopes are better suited for larger lesions and when imaging for extraluminal pathology is required.

Performing EUS from inside the stomach can take some time to master because factors such as gastric motility, retained gastric bubbles or debris, respiratory motion, and the non-uniform contour of the stomach can all impact image acquisition and quality. When evaluating large, mobile, pedunculated gastric polyps, it can be difficult to obtain EUS images of

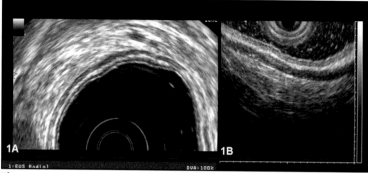

Figure 10-1. EUS of normal gastric wall. (A) Normal 5-layer gastric wall pattern seen using radial echoendoscope. Layer 1, Interface layer at the "Superficial" mucosa (Hyperechoic/Bright). Layer 2, "Deep" mucosa (Hypoechoic/Dark). Layer 3, Submucosa (Hyperechoic/Bright). Layer 4, Muscularis propria (Hypoechoic/Dark). Layer 5, Subserosa/serosa (Hyperechoic/Bright). (B) Higher resolution using a high-frequency ultrasound miniprobe. In this example, 7 echolayers can be distinguished.

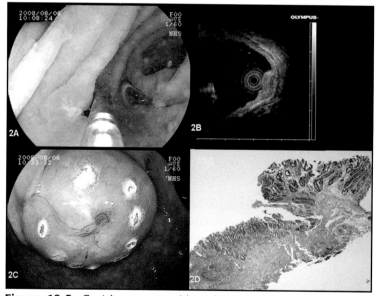

Figure 10-2. Gastric cancer with submucosal involvement (T1). (A) Small ulcerated lesion in gastric antrum during evaluation with high-frequency ultrasound miniprobe. (B) EUS appearance demonstrates area of ulceration with irregular contour and involvement of the submucosa (layer 3) with an intact muscularis propria (layer 4). (C) Appearance after marking the borders of the lesion and "lifting" with submucosal saline. (D) Histological appearance of lesion confirmed invasion the submucosa.

the base of the stalk at the point of insertion into the gastric wall; often, the stalk is compressed against the adjacent gastric mucosa, which can lead to EUS errors. Various techniques can help to minimize some of these technical challenges. Instillation of de-aerated water into the gastric lumen helps remove bubbles and debris and provides acoustic coupling for better image quality (elevating the head of the bed helps minimize aspiration of the instilled water). It may also cause pedunculated polyps to "float," facilitating EUS of the stalk.

I generally recommend that the examination be performed in a series of steps to maximize the quality of the examination. First, place the ultrasound transducer in close proximity to the distal margin of the tumor and slowly pull the scope proximally to the proximal margin of the tumor, keeping the transducer relatively close and as perpendicular as possible to the mass. This facilitates T-staging. Then, starting from the duodenal bulb, perform a "pull back" to the esophagogastric junction, keeping the transducer relatively centered in the stomach. This enables a global evaluation for perigastric lymph nodes or regional pathology. Because the depth of radial EUS imaging is only 5 to 7 cm, more distant pathology may be missed by this pull-back (eg, lymph nodes along the greater curvature of the stomach, some liver lesions). These areas can then be interrogated further, as needed, by additional "pull-backs" with the endoscope tip deflected toward the liver, the greater curvature, and the lesser curvature.

Role of Endoscopic Ultrasound in Differentiating Non-Neoplastic and Neoplastic Gastric Pathology

In most cases, diagnosing gastric malignancy with upper endoscopy and forceps biopsy is straightforward. However, at times, the diagnosis can be difficult to make, as with scirrhous gastric carcinomas that infiltrate within the gastric wall, produce "thickened gastric folds," and are not infrequently associated with negative forceps biopsies. EUS can help distinguish scirrhous carcinomas from other benign or malignant causes of thickened folds (eg, severe gastritis, Menetrier's disease, lymphoma). In general, the gastric wall is considered thickened when total wall thickness exceeds approximately 3 to 4 mm. Diffuse, widespread thickening that is limited to the first 2 echolayers (the "superficial" and "deep" mucosa) is almost always attributable to a benign process, such as hypertrophic gastritis. Conversely, the third and/or fourth echolayers (the submucosa and muscularis propria) are typically also thickened in patients with a malignant cause of "thickened folds." With scirrhous carcinomas, the 5-echolayer wall pattern is often still recognizable despite the infiltrating carcinoma (Figure 10-3), whereas infiltrating lymphomas tend to obliterate the echolayer pattern, replacing them with hypoechoic (dark) tumor tissue. Despite these generalizations, when faced with the "thickened" folds dilemma, one can frequently obtain diagnostic samples by doing FNA of the gastric wall and (if needed after FNA) performing a focal endoscopic resection of the thickened fold. EUS-FNA also helps differentiate other gastric abnormalities, such as leiomyomas, carcinoids, gastrointestinal stromal tumors (GIST), heterotopic pancreas (pancreatic rest), and not infrequently identifying extrinsic compression caused by the gallbladder, liver, or spleen.

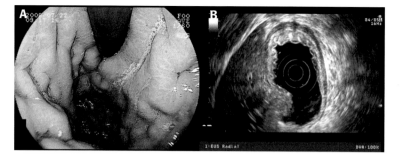

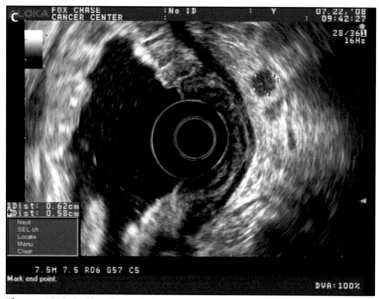

Figure 10-3. Infiltrative scirrhous adenocarcinoma of the gastric body ("linitis plastica"). (A) Endoscopic view (retroflexed) shows abnormally thickened gastric folds. (B) EUS appearance demonstrates thickening of the gastric wall, including the muscularis propria (layer 4), with relative *preservation* of the 5-layer gastric wall pattern. Note the preferential thickening of the greater curvature (top half of image); most of the lesser curvature appears normal. (C) Abnormal perigastric lymph node (round, hypoechoic, well-demarcated borders. Surgical gastrectomy confirmed a T2N1 infiltrating gastric carcinoma (using AJCC, 6th edition criteria).

Endoscopic Ultrasound
for Staging of Gastric Adenocarcinoma

The first imaging study for a patient with newly diagnosed adenocarcinoma should be cross-sectional imaging with computerized tomography (CT) scan to evaluate for distant metastatic disease. If findings consistent with metastatic disease are identified, subsequent imaging with EUS is unnecessary unless EUS-FNA is requested to obtain confirmatory tissue (eg, FNA of liver lesions, distant lymphadenopathy). EUS should be considered if no evidence of metastatic disease is identified on cross-sectional imaging. It remains unclear whether pretreatment EUS should be performed routinely in patients with gastric cancer. A flow diagram in the current NCCN guidelines (National Comprehensive Cancer Network) lists EUS as "optional," although a subsequent text section of the guidelines describes EUS as "indicated for assessing depth of tumor invasion."[1] EUS for gastric cancer is frequently (though not universally) performed at my institution because it can facilitate treatment decisions, such as whether to administer neoadjuvant (preoperative) chemotherapy or attempt endoscopic resection for dysplastic lesions or early stage (T1) cancers. EUS may also be required to assess eligibility for enrollment in clinical trials.

There are 2 main gastric cancer staging systems: the Japanese Gastric Cancer Association system and the American Joint Committee on Cancer/International Union Against Cancer (AJCC/UICC) staging system. The latter uses a TNM classification schema and is the primary system used in the United States.[2] The 2010 AJCC staging definitions (7th edition) are shown in Tables 10-1 and 10-2. There are several noteworthy changes compared to the prior 6th edition that practicing endosonographers should adopt. For example, tumors arising from 5 cm or less from the esophagogastric junction and crossing the esophagogastric junction should now be staged using the TNM system for esophageal adenocarcinoma. In addition, there are modifications in the tumor (T) staging (ie, subdividing T1 cancers into T1a and T1b) and the nodal (N) staging, which impact EUS staging.

EUS T-stage and N-stage accuracy rates reported for gastric cancers range from 68% to 92% (mean: 80%) and 50% to 100% (mean: 72%), respectively. EUS appears least accurate for T2 cancers, primarily because of over-staging (labeling it as a T3 lesion erroneously), which may occur for several reasons, especially peritumoral inflammation. The endosonographic appearance of T2 and T3 tumors may also differ depending on the macroscopic appearance of the tumor. Cancers with a "medullary"-type growth pattern have a better demarcated border and a homogeneous hypoechoic internal pattern, whereas those with scirrhous-type growth patterns tend to have an undefined border and heterogeneous internal echo. Recognition of the different EUS appearances of T2 and T3 medullary versus scirrhous carcinomas may improve the accuracy of EUS.[3] Regarding N-staging, it can be difficult to determine whether a lymph node is malignant or benign based solely on EUS appearance. EUS features suggestive of malignancy are shown in Table 10-3. The presence of all 4 features is greater than 80% predictive of malignancy, though only approximately 25% of malignant lymph nodes have all 4 features. Conversely, nonmalignant lymph nodes often have one or more of these characteristics.

Compared to cross-sectional imaging (CT, MRI), EUS has historically been accepted as more reliable for T-staging and comparable for local N-staging, though enhancements in CT and MRI technology continue to improve their accuracy. FNA of suspicious nodes and extra-gastric lesions (eg, liver lesions, ascites) enhances the value of EUS, and EUS should be performed when tissue confirmation of malignancy will impact clinical management. Care should be used to avoid traversing the primary tumor while performing FNA, to avoid tumor seeding.

Table 10-1

American Joint Committee on Cancer/International Union Against Cancer Staging System for Gastric Adenocarcinoma

Primary Tumor (T)	
TX	Primary tumor cannot be assessed
T0	No evidence of primary tumor
Tis	Carcinoma in situ: intraepithelial tumor without invasion of the lamina propria
T1	Tumor invades lamina propria, muscularis mucosae, or submucosa
T1a	Tumor invades lamina propria or muscularis mucosae
T1b	Tumor invades submucosa
T2	Tumor invades muscularis propria*
T3	Tumor penetrates subserosal connective tissue without invasion of visceral peritoneum or adjacent structures**,***
T4	Tumor invades serosa (visceral peritoneum) or adjacent structures**,***
T4a	Tumor invades serosa (visceral peritoneum)
T4b	Tumor invades adjacent structures

*Note: A tumor may penetrate the muscularis propria with extension into the gastrocolic or gastrohepatic ligaments, or into the greater or lesser omentum, without perforation of the visceral peritoneum covering these structures. In this case, the tumor is classified T3. If there is perforation of the visceral peritoneum covering the gastric ligaments or the omentum, the tumor should be classified T4.

**The adjacent structures of the stomach include the spleen, transverse colon, liver, diaphragm, pancreas, abdominal wall, adrenal gland, kidney, small intestine, and retroperitoneum.

***Intramural extension to the deodenum or esophagus is classified by the depth of the greatest invasion in any of these sites, including the stomach.

Regional Lymph Nodes (N)	
NX	Regional lymph node(s) cannot be assessed
N0	No regional lymph node metastasis*
N1	Metastasis in 1 to 2 regional lymph nodes
N2	Metastasis in 3 to 6 regional lymph nodes
N3	Metastasis in 7 or more regional lymph nodes
N3a	Metastasis in 7 to 15 regional lymph nodes
N3b	Metastasis in 16 or more regional lymph nodes

*Note: A designation of pN0 should be used if all examined lymph nodes are negative, regardless of the total number removed and examined.

Distant Metastasis (M)	
M0	No distant metastasis
M1	Distant metastasis

Table 10-2

American Joint Committee on Cancer/International Union Against Cancer Staging System for Gastric Adenocarcinoma

Anatomic Stage/Prognostic Groups			
Stage 0	Tis	N0	M0
Stage IA	T1	N0	M0
Stage IB	T2	N0	M0
	T1	N1	M0
Stage IIA	T3	N0	M0
	T2	N1	M0
	T1	N2	M0
Stage IIB	T4a	N0	M0
	T3	N1	M0
	T2	N2	M0
	TI	N3	M0
Stage IIIA	T4a	N1	M0
	T3	N2	M0
	T2	N3	M0
Stage IIIB	T4b	N0	M0
	T4b	N1	M0
	T4a	N2	M0
	T3	N3	M0
Stage IIIC	T4b	N2	M0
	T4b	N3	M0
	T4a	N3	M0
Stage IV	Any T	Any N	M1

Reprinted with the permission of the American Joint Committee on Cancer (AJCC), Chicago, Illinois. The original source for this material is the *AJCC Cancer Staging Manual, Seventh Edition* (2010) published by Springer Science and Business Media LLC, www.springer.com. Stomach. In: Edge SE, Byrd DR, Carducci MA, Compton CC, eds. *AJCC Cancer Staging Manual.* 7th ed. New York, NY: Springer; 2010:117-126.

Table 10-3
Endoscopic Ultrasound Characteristics of Malignant versus Benign Lymph Nodes

Malignant	Benign
Round or oval	Flat, triangular, "draping"
Homogeneous, hypoechoic	Heterogeneous, centrally hyperechoic
Sharp borders (well-defined)	Poorly defined borders ('fuzzy')
Size >10 mm	Size <10 mm
	Presence of intact intra-nodal vasculature

References

1. National Comprehensive Cancer Network. NCCN practice guidelines in oncology: gastric cancer v.2.2010. http://www.nccn.org/professionals/physician_gls/PDF/gastric.pdf. Accessed April 20, 2010.
2. Stomach. In: Edge SE, Byrd DR, Carducci MA, Compton CC, eds. *AJCC Cancer Staging Manual.* 7th ed. New York, NY: Springer; 2010:117-126.
3. Kida M. EUS in gastric cancer. In: Hawes RH, Fockens P, eds. *Endosonography.* Philadelphia, PA: Saunders Elsevier; 2006:111-126.

How Is Tumor-Related Bleeding From Gastric Cancers Best Approached?

Jeffrey L. Tokar, MD

Only 25% to 40% of patients with gastric carcinoma will have localized disease at diagnosis and will be eligible for potentially curative surgical resection.[1] Bleeding, pain, and obstructive symptoms (dysphagia, nausea, vomiting) are common in patients with advanced cancers and can significantly impact quality of life. Tumor bleeding, whether overt (ie, melena, hematesis) or occult (ie, chronic iron-deficiency anemia), can result in interruptions in chemotherapy treatment, fatigue, dyspnea, frequent hospitalizations or blood transfusions, and exacerbation of pre-existing cardiopulmonary comorbidities. From the perspective of the on-call gastroenterologist, massive and/or hemodynamically unstable bleeding from gastric carcinoma is distinctly uncommon, and the need to perform emergent endoscopic intervention is exceedingly rare. Medical oncologists may be particularly concerned about tumor bleeding, particularly when they plan to use cancer therapies that can either exacerbate anemia or cause iatrogenic gastrointestinal hemorrhage (eg, bevacizumab).

According to the National Comprehensive Cancer Network's "principles of best supportive care," gastric cancer patients with acute bleeding should undergo prompt endoscopic assessment with endoscopic hemostatic interventions "appropriate to the findings." When endoscopic hemostasis cannot be achieved, angiographic embolization techniques by the interventional radiology team may be considered, although these sometimes come with the risk of ischemic injury to the gastric wall. External beam radiation is the third recommended treatment and is advocated for patients with chronic tumor bleeding.[2] In my opinion, any therapy for tumor bleeding should only be offered to patients with clinically significant bleeding because all forms of therapy have limitations and the potential for complications.

Figure 11-1. Endoscopic view of gastric malignancy with diffuse, active mucosal bleeding before endoscopic therapy (left) and after endoscopic therapy with argon plasma coagulation (right).

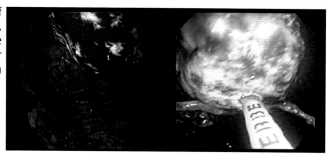

Endoscopic Therapy for Gastric Cancer Bleeding

Not infrequently, nontumor-related causes of bleeding (eg, peptic ulcer disease, angio-ectasias) are identified in patients known to have gastric cancer and should be sought and treated rather than assuming the patient has tumor bleeding. There is a relative dearth of studies *specific* to this clinical entity. Large prospective trials of endoscopic therapy (ET) are lacking; most of the available information comes from small numbers of patients with tumor bleeding included in larger cohorts undergoing ET for either (1) hemostasis of a wide variety of bleeding etiologies (not only tumor bleeding) or for (2) "tumor palliation" (tumor debulking to prevent obstruction in most cases; fewer patients were treated for control of tumor bleeding).

Published reports on laser photocoagulation suggest that initial control of tumor bleed-ing can be achieved in 65% to 95% of patients after one or more treatment sessions, but rebleeding rates are as high as 80%. Laser therapy is expensive, unwieldy, and relatively time consuming.

Argon plasma coagulation (APC) has tumor ablation capabilities comparable to laser photocoagulation, and the newer electrosurgical generators provide improved power regu-lation and a broader range of settings, allowing greater control of the energy delivered to tumor tissue and some degree of "tailoring" of the thermal effect to fit the clinical situation. APC is currently my preferred endoscopic option for patients with diffuse mucosal bleed-ing from tumor surfaces (Figure 11-1). I tend to avoid "contact" methods of thermal ablation (eg, bipolar electrocoagulation, heater probe) in these cases because the cauterized tissue "sticks" to the probe, which then requires repetitive cleaning, increasing the duration of the procedure. It is important to remember that APC will be less effective if there is a layer of blood on the target tissue because APC tends to coagulate blood and produce a carbonated "eschar" that may prevent the plasma arc from contacting the tumor.

For superficial, nonbulky tumors, I "paint" the surface of the tumor using a rapid pulsed APC mode, which can achieve hemostasis with limited depth of injury. For larger, bulky tumors that may benefit from debulking, I may begin with a rapid superficial pulsed mode but eventually switch to a more ablative mode. If the surface of the tumor becomes desiccated and charred, mechanical removal of surface eschar exposes deeper tumor that can then be fulgurated. Iatrogenic bleeding can occur and may require addi-tional or alternative interventions. My personal experience has been that APC hemostasis can be achieved in most patients with 1 to 3 treatment sessions and usually does not require extensive tumor debulking, but control of bleeding is rarely permanent.

Mechanical methods (endoscopic clips, ligating loops) for hemostasis in this setting have been used in a limited manner. Published case reports/series of successful mechanical hemostasis in this setting are available, but there are few large-scale data on these devices in this setting.

Several other novel endoscopic modalities deserve mention (though none are currently recommended for routine use). A recent pilot study of radiofrequency energy delivered directly into rectal cancers via specially designed radiofrequency energy probes achieved effective tumor ablation and hemostasis. Cryospray ablation induces capillary injury and microthrombus formation; the resulting microcirculatory stasis may be effective for tumor bleeding. Ankaferd Blood Stopper (Ankaferd Health Products, Ltd, Istanbul, Turkey) is a hemostatic herbal extract derived from 5 different plants (*Thymus vulgaris, Glycyrrhiza glabra, Vitis vinifera, Alpinia officinarum,* and *Urtica dioica*) that was recently approved in Turkey for postsurgical and postdental bleeding. It rapidly (<1 second) promotes formation of a specific protein network, which facilitates hemostasis as demonstrated in animal models and limited human experience.[3] Future studies of ABS for control of gastrointestinal (GI) bleeding in humans are anticipated. Case reports of injecting various sclerosants and tissue adhesives directly into tumors for debulking, including interventional endoscopic ultrasound (I-EUS)-guided fine-needle injection into neoplasms, have been published but are experimental.

Transcatheter Arterial Embolization for Gastric Cancer Bleeding

While the efficacy of transcatheter arterial embolization (TCE) for upper GI bleeding not amenable to endoscopic therapy is well described, there are relatively few published data regarding embolization for gastric cancer bleeding *specifically.* In one recent retrospective study from Korea, 23 gastric cancer patients with acute bleeding underwent angiographic intervention.[4] Approximately half of these patients were either not amenable to endoscopic therapy or had recurrent or continued bleeding after endoscopic interventions. Super-selective TCE using microcatheters and gelatin sponge particles, micro-coils, or glue achieved clinical hemostasis in 6 of 8 patients (75%) with active bleeding, and 3 of 7 patients (43%) with tumor blush but no active bleeding on angiography. TCE can also play a role when active bleeding is not identified.

Radiotherapy for Palliation of Gastric Cancer Bleeding

External beam radiotherapy (ERT) is primarily used concurrently with chemotherapy for adjuvant (and, in some institutions, neoadjuvant) therapy for locally advanced gastric cancers. The ability of ERT to decrease total tumor volume and to potentially contribute to an overall survival advantage, when combined with chemotherapy, is an advantage of ERT over ET and TCE. Most patients with *metastatic* gastric cancer are treated with chemotherapy alone, reserving ERT for palliation of tumor-related complications

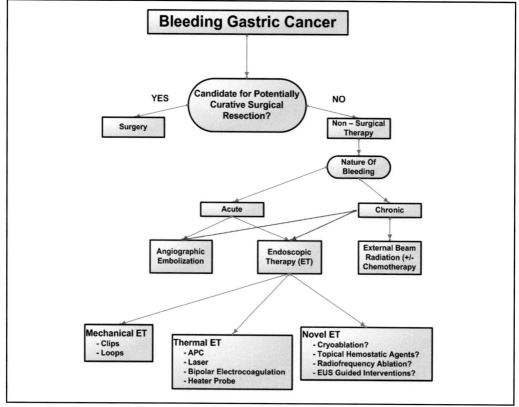

Figure 11-2. Flow chart depicting a general approach to management of bleeding from gastric cancer.

(eg, pain, obstruction, and bleeding). However, the body of literature assessing the hemostatic benefit of ERT *specifically* for gastric cancer bleeding is limited to small series in which variable dose-fractionation regimens were used (regimens from 30 Gy in 10 fractions to 54 Gy in 30 fractions are often used). Durable control of tumor bleeding can be achieved in most patients (approximately 55% to 75%). Median durations of hemostasis as high as 11 to 12 months have been reported.[5,6]

In a recent series in which ERT achieved hemostasis in 73% of 30 patients with transfusion-requiring gastric cancer bleeding, patients who had received concurrent chemotherapy with ERT appeared to have lower re-bleeding rates than those receiving ERT alone.[7] In my experience, the durability of ERT hemostasis for diffuse mucosal tumor bleeding exceeds that of endoscopic ablation, and ERT should be considered in nonacute tumor bleeding in patients who are more likely to recognize the benefit (ie, adequate life expectancy). ERT has limitations, however, including a limited role in acute active GI bleeding, plus its potential to cause gastritis, ulcers, or hypochlorhydria (if a significant parietal cell volume is irradiated). These sequelae can cause or exacerbate nausea, vomiting, and dyspepsia/pain and may induce nontumor-related bleeding.

Unfortunately, despite best supportive care for patients with advanced unresectable gastric cancer, the prognosis is poor.[7] Management of this challenging cohort of patients requires judicious clinical decision making and a multidisciplinary approach. My basic algorithm to gastric cancer bleeding is summarized in Figure 11-2.

References

1. Perez CA. *Principles and Practice of Radiation Oncology.* 4th ed. Philadelphia, PA: Lippincott Williams & Wilkins; 2004.
2. National Comprehensive Cancer Network. NCCN practice guidelines in oncology: gastric cancer v.2.2010. http://www.nccn.org/professionals/physician_gls/PDF/gastric.pdf. Accessed April 20, 2010.
3. Turhan N, Kurt M, Shorbagi A, Akdogan M, Haznedaroglu IC. Topical Ankaferd Blood Stopper administration to bleeding gastrointestinal carcinomas decreases tumor vascularization. *Am J Gastroenterol.* 2009;104(11):2874-2877.
4. Lee HJ, Shin JH, Yoon HK, et al. Transcatheter arterial embolization in gastric cancer patients with acute bleeding. *Eur Radiol.* 2009;19(4):960-965.
5. Kim MM, Rana V, Janjan NA, et al. Clinical benefit of palliative radiation therapy in advanced gastric cancer. *Acta Oncol.* 2008;47(3):421-427.
6. Tey J, Back MF, Shakespeare TP, et al. The role of palliative radiation therapy in symptomatic locally advanced gastric cancer. *Int J Radiat Oncol Biol Phys.* 2007;67(2):385-388.
7. Asakura H, Hashimoto T, Harada H, et al. Palliative radiotherapy for bleeding from advanced gastric cancer: is a schedule of 30 Gy in 10 fractions adequate? *J Cancer Res Clin Oncol.* 2011;137(1):125-130.

WHAT IS LINITIS PLASTICA, AND HOW DOES ITS DEVELOPMENT AFFECT THE MANAGEMENT AND PROGNOSIS OF PATIENTS WITH GASTRIC CANCER?

Caroline R. Tadros, MD

Linitis plastica (LP) refers to anaplastic carcinoma that is characterized by diffuse intramural infiltration. This results in wall thickening and decreased volume of a hollow viscous. It can occur throughout the gastrointestinal (GI) tract; however, the stomach is the most commonly affected organ.[1,2] It has been reported to occur in 3% to 19% of all gastric carcinomas[1] (Figure 12-1).

LP typically arises from the lower third of the mucosa and is associated with an extensive desmoplastic reaction in the submucosa.[1] Fibrosis can also be found within the subserosa and muscularis due to the increased deposition of types I and IV collagen.[1] Despite the degree of fibrosis, the architecture of the wall layers remains intact.[1,2] The 2 most common cell types noted in LP are signet-ring and poorly differentiated adenocarcinoma.[1]

LP is associated with adenomatous polyposis coli (APC) gene mutations and modified expression of class II (HLA-DR) antigens on tumor cells.[2] LP has also been associated with autosomal dominant germline mutation in the E-cadherin gene (CDH1). Cadherins (calcium-dependent adhesion molecules) are located on the surface of cells and allow cells to adhere to one another. The mutation in CDH1 results in modified expression of cadherins on the surface of fibroblasts and signet cells. This results in a loss of adhesiveness and may allow for tumor to develop within the dense stromal reaction.[2,3]

The antrum and pylorus are the most common gastric sites of LP, and the rate of proximal spread to the gastric body varies. The fundus is not typically involved.[1] LP is an aggressive infiltrative process and therefore has a propensity to involve the entire stomach, invade the serosa, metastasize to lymph nodes, and seed the peritoneum.[1,4]

Figure 12-1. Endoscopic image of a patient with linitis plastica type cancer. Note universal wall thickening and luminal narrowing. (Reprinted with permission of Douglas G. Adler, MD.)

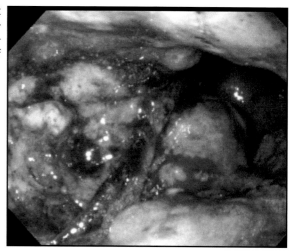

Patients with LP are frequently diagnosed at an advanced stage due to the lack of signs or symptoms early on in the course of the disease. The most common symptoms include epigastric pain, progressive dysphagia to solids and liquids, anorexia, and weight loss. Patients rarely present with hematemesis, perforation, or signs of gastric outlet obstruction. Pseudoachalasia has also been associated with LP when there is infiltration of the cardia.[1] Physical examination may reveal a lump in the epigastrum but is often unremarkable. Endoscopic evaluation may reveal thickened gastric folds with luminal narrowing, nodular mucosa with red lesions, or pyloric stenosis. In the setting of pseudoachalasia, esophageal dilation may be noted, and resistance to passage of the endoscope may be encountered at the GE junction.[1] Differential diagnosis includes lymphoma, Menetier's gastritis, amyloidosis, lymphoid hyperplasia, sarcoidosis, tuberculosis, Crohn's disease, CMV gastritis, corrosive gastritis, and idiopathic fibrosing hypertrophic gastritis.[1,5,6]

The diagnosis of LP can be difficult to make with routine endoscopic biopsies, because the neoplastic process occurs deep to the mucosa. Therefore, the mucosal surface can still appear normal. The variation in cell density within the desmoplastic reaction can also lead to false negative biopsies.[3] Diathermic snares have been used in order to obtain deeper histological samples; however, due to the increased risk of hemorrhage and perforation, "stacked" forcep biopsies have been recommended for initial evaluation.[1]

Endoscopic ultrasound (EUS) and computed tomography (CT) are instrumental in the diagnosis and staging of LP. Thickening of the gastric wall to more than 1 cm is suggestive of LP, but is not diagnostic. EUS provides a more detailed evaluation of the gastric wall layers and nodal disease and allows for FNA to establish the diagnosis[1] (Figure 12-2).

The prognosis of LP is extremely poor due to the fact that it has a propensity to seed the peritoneum. Extensive surgical resection is required for cure; however, there remains debate as to the optimal surgical approach. In 1988, Furukawa and colleagues recommended radical surgery, which also included resection of the spleen, pancreatic body and tail, transverse colon, left adrenal, and gallbladder with extensive lymphadenectomy. This approach demonstrated a significant decrease in local regional recurrence at 3 years for both T2 and T3 lesions and was not associated with increased morbidity and mortality.[2] In

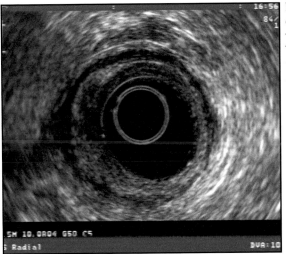

Figure 12-2. A 7.5-MHz EUS image of circumferential mucosal and submucosal thickening in a patient with linitis plastica. The muscularis propria deep to the submucosal is also thickened and irregular, and this can be due to either direct tumor involvement or peritumoral inflammation. (Reprinted with permission of Douglas G. Adler, MD.)

1999, Hamy and coworkers recommend total gastrectomy with a D1 or D2 nodal resection due to the infiltrative nature of LP. However, Kodera and colleagues subsequently demonstrated that disseminated cancer cells are present in peritoneal washings at the time of laparotomy in up to 70% to 80% of patients referred for resection, arguing against extensive resection.[1,4] In 2008, Kodera and colleagues found that patients with more than 16 positive lymph nodes had a worse prognosis, as this correlated with bony metastases. Hence, staging laparoscopy is typically performed prior to surgical resection to rule out peritoneal and/or extensive nodal involvement.

Chemotherapy with an oral fluoropyrimidine (TS-1) has been shown to prolong survival in patients with unresectable LP. The median survival in patients receiving TS-1 was 402 days, as opposed to 213 days seen in patients receiving standard chemotherapy with 5-fluorouracil, cisplatin, methotrexate, and mitomycin-C. The optimal management of LP remains controversial. Many authors propose that chemotherapy should be the cornerstone of management, while others recommend a combination of chemotherapy (adjuvant systemic and/or intra-peritoneal, or chemohyperthermia) and radical surgery.[1]

Conclusion

LP is a diffuse anaplastic carcinoma within a hollow viscous that is characterized by an intense desmoplastic response. There appears to be a genetic component as familial clustering has been observed, and there is a strong association with the APC gene and germline mutations, which lead to truncated formation of e-cadherin. The prognosis is poor as patients are often unresectable at the time of diagnosis. LP is particularly aggressive with a high rate of lymph node metastases and peritoneal seeding. The diagnosis can be challenging as symptoms are vague in the early stages of disease. Because the neoplastic process occurs submucosally, routine endoscopy may be unrevealing. A combination of CT and EUS may be more appropriate in high-risk patients. There is debate regarding the management of these patients; however, given that most patients have evidence of peritoneal involvement at the time of laparoscopy, a combination of chemotherapy and surgery seems reasonable. Because there seems to be a genetic component, identifying patients at high risk for LP and enrolling them in aggressive screening programs should be considered.

References

1. Mastoraki A, Papanikolaou IS, Sakorfas G, Safioleas M. Facing the challenge of managing linitis plastic— Review of the literature. *Hepatogastroenterology*. 2009;56(96):1773-1778.
2. Hamy A, Letessier E, Bizouarn P, et al. Study of survival and prognostic factors in patients undergoing resection for gastric linitis plastica: A review of 86 cases. *Int Surg*. 1999;84(4):337-343.
3. Dussaulx-Garin L, Blayau M, Pagenault M, et al. A new mutation of E-cadherin gene in familial gastric linitis plastica cancer with extra-digestive dissemination. *Eur J Gastroenterol Hepatol*. 2001;13(6):711-715.
4. Kodera Y, Ito S, Mochizuki Y, et al. The number of metastatic lymph nodes is a significant risk factor for bone metastasis and poor outcome after surgery for linitis plastica-type gastric carcinoma. *World J Surg*. 2008;32(9):2015-2020.
5. Talukdar R, Khanna S, Saikia N, Vij JC. Gastric tuberculosis presenting as linitis plastica: a case report and review of the literature. *Eur J Gastroenterol Hepatol*. 2006;18(3):299-303.
6. Terada T. Idiopathic fibrosing hypertrophic gastritis: a new entity that mimics linitis plastica carcinoma. *Endoscopy*. 2009;41(Suppl 2):E90.

A 42-Year-Old Woman Has an Esophago-gastroduodenoscopy for Dyspepsia. A 2-cm Submucosal Lesion in the Proximal Stomach Is Seen. How Should This Lesion Be Further Evaluated and Treated?

Robert C. Wrona, MD and Robert E. Glasgow, MD

The incidence of submucosal lesions of the stomach is approximately 0.36% on routine esophagogastroduodenoscopy (EGD) performed for abdominal pain[1] (Figure 13-1). The true incidence of these lesions, however, is unknown as most submucosal lesions are asymptomatic and discovered incidentally at autopsy, surgery, or during diagnostic procedures. The differential diagnosis of a submucosal lesion includes an extramural tumor, benign mesenchymal tumors (including leiomyomas, schwannomas, neurofibromas, hemangiomas, lymphangiomas, lipomas, and heterotopic pancreas), and malignant tumors (including leiomyosarcoma, metastases, Kaposi's sarcoma, and gastrointestinal stromal tumor [GIST]).

Identification of a submucosal lesion on routine endoscopy should be followed by endoscopic ultrasound (EUS) to confirm an intramural source (Figure 13-2). EUS is used to measure the tumor's size for further treatment planning, to evaluate for concerning characteristics of malignancy (size greater than approximately 3 cm, an irregular border, echogenic foci, cystic spaces, and malignant-appearing lymph nodes), and to evaluate for gastric wall layer of origin.

Further diagnostic testing to evaluate a submucosal lesion of the stomach may include fine needle aspiration via endoscopic ultrasound (which is preferred over percutaneous biopsy, which has the potential of tumor seeding). Conventional mucosal biopsy with routine endoscopy is inadequate unless the gastric mucosa is ulcerated. The efficacy of

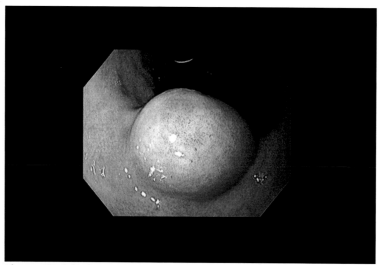

Figure 13-1. Endoscopic appearance of a 2-cm (GIST).

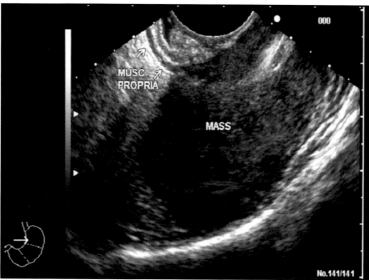

Figure 13-2. Endoscopic ultrasound appearance of a 2-cm GIST. Note communication of the lesion with the muscularis propria (arrow).

fine-needle aspiration with endoscopic ultrasound is controversial. Sensitivities reported in the literature range from 58% to 91% and are largely dependent on getting enough tissue to characterize the lesion as a spindle cell tumor and to provide ample tissue for immunohistochemistry.[2-4] Moreover, according to guidelines from the National Comprehensive Cancer Network (NCCN), any preoperative biopsy of a submucosal lesion carries significant risks of hemorrhage and seeding and may not be appropriate if the tumor is easily resectable.[5] Endoscopic ultrasound-guided fine-needle aspiration, however, should be performed with large lesions in which preoperative chemotherapy with imatinib may be considered.

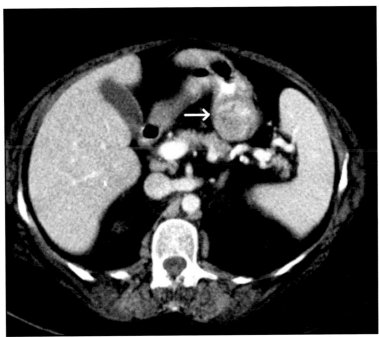

Figure 13-3. Computed tomography scan demonstrating a 2-cm GIST (arrow).

CT scan alone is not reliable in characterizing a submucosal tumor of the stomach, although the finding of an exophytic, hypervascular mass is suggestive of a gastrointestinal stromal tumor (Figure 13-3). CT scan is useful for delineating lesion size, relation to adjacent organs, and the presence of metastases and is, therefore, a useful adjunct for staging, surgical planning, and assessing response to therapy. All patients with a submucosal gastric lesion where there is a suspicion of GIST should undergo an abdominal CT scan to help guide further treatment even if EUS has been performed. Similarly, conventional chest imaging should be performed to evaluate for thoracic metastases.

The most common malignant submucosal or mesenchymal lesion of the gastrointestinal tract is a GIST, affecting approximately 6000 patients per year. GISTs arise from the interstitial cells of Cajal via activating mutations in one of the receptor protein tyrosine kinases (KIT, also called CD-117). Approximately 95% of GISTs express KIT. Another 5% express mutations in the platelet derived growth factor alpha (PDGFA) genes and are KIT negative. Approximately, 60% of GISTs occur in the stomach. The presentation of a patient with a GIST is highly variable, spanning the spectrum from asymptomatic to symptoms of early satiety, bleeding, nausea, bloating, or fatigue from anemia to a palpable abdominal mass. As is the case in this patient, small lesions are almost always asymptomatic and found incidentally. If fine-needle aspiration under endoscopic ultrasound is performed, the pathologic evaluation should include mitotic count, immunohistochemistry for cd34 and cd117, and molecular genetic analysis for PDGFA and KIT mutations.

In patients with a GIST, median age at diagnosis is 63 with a slight preponderance in men. The median size of GISTs is 6 cm. At diagnosis, 53% of cases of GIST were staged as localized, 19% regional, and 23% distant spread with the remaining 5% unstaged.[6] The liver and peritoneal cavity are the most common locations of metastases. Pulmonary and extra-abdominal disease is seen in advanced cases.

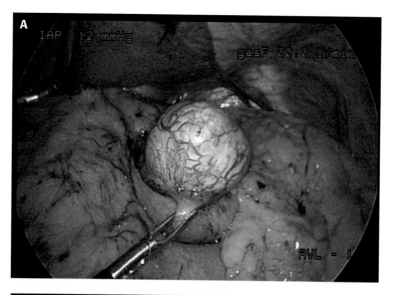

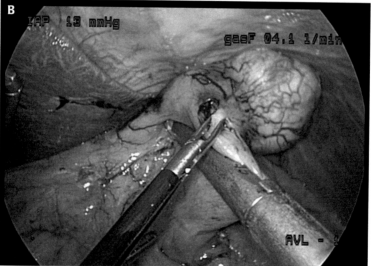

Figure 13-4. (A) Laparoscopic appearance of a GIST. (B) Laparoscopic wedge resection of GIST.

Any patient with a submucosal lesion that may be a GIST should be considered for surgical resection, which not only confirms the diagnosis but provides the primary therapy and allows for risk stratification by means of pathologic analysis. Surgical therapy should achieve negative margins via wedge or segmental resection. Extended anatomic resections with extensive lymph node dissection are not indicated. Laparoscopic surgery is appropriate in the treatment of GISTs, provided oncologic principles are maintained, and is the preferred approach for small lesions where a nonanatomic resection is feasible (Figure 13-4). In patients who underwent complete primary resection, recurrence-free survival was 83%, 75%, and 63% at 1, 2, and 5 years, respectively. On multivariate analysis, recurrence was predicted by 5 or more mitoses/50 high-power fields, tumor size of 10 cm or larger, and tumor location (with patients having small bowel GIST doing the worst).[7]

Table 13-1

Risk Analysis for Gastrointestinal Stromal Tumor

Risk	Size	Mitotic Rate
High	Any size	> 10/50 HPF
	> 10 cm	Any rate
	> 5 cm	> 5/50 HPF
Intermediate	5 to 10 cm	< 5/50 HPF
	< 5 cm	6 to 10/50 HPF
Low	2 to 5 cm	< 5/50 HPF
Very low	< 2 cm	< 5/50 HPF

Recently, a nomogram has been developed to aid in predicting risk of recurrence, including smaller lesions.[8] If surgical resection would cause considerable morbidity at initial evaluation, neoadjuvant imatinib should be considered to reduce tumor size and allow for a less extensive resection to achieve negative margins.

The NCCN has suggested that, for GISTs less than 2 cm, observation with repeat endoscopic ultrasound surveillance every 6 to 12 months is acceptable, provided the patient has been fully informed of the risks and benefits.[5] The rationale for this approach is the extremely low risk of metastatic potential and tumor size progression in this group. This strategy, however, does require diagnostic fine-needle aspiration biopsy. If the lesion has an irregular border, cystic spaces, ulceration, echogenic foci, or heterogeneity, surgical resection is mandated. EUS also provides the best method of size measurement as increasing size would be an absolute indication for surgical resection.

According to the NCCN, complete resection of GISTs is possible in approximately 85% of patients with primary tumors, and 50% of these patients will develop recurrence or metastasis following complete resection.[5] The biggest development in the ongoing treatment of GISTs postoperatively has been identification of specific tyrosine inhibitors, such as imatinib, which have demonstrated efficacy in extending survival in GIST patients. Imatinib and newer-generation tyrosine inhibitors should be considered in all patients considered to have high-risk lesions either preoperatively to improve the potential for a R0 resection or as adjunctive treatment for intermediate or high-risk lesions (Table 13-1). Small lesions only rarely display unfavorable histology or mitotic activity and, therefore, seldom require adjuvant treatment with a tyrosine kinase inhibitor. These small lesions are almost always resectable.

Follow-up of all GIST patients after surgical resection includes a history and physical as well as abdominal/pelvic CT every 3 to 6 months for the first 3 to 5 years, then annually. Recurrence warrants referral to a medical oncologist and discussion at a multidisciplinary soft-tissue sarcoma tumor board with experience in managing GIST patients for consideration of surgical resection and adjuvant therapy.

References

1. Hedenbro JL, Ekelund M, Wetterberg P. Endoscopic diagnosis of submucosal gastric lesions. The results after routine endoscopy. *Surg Endosc.* 1991;5(1):20-23.
2. Hoda KM, Rodriguez SA, Faigel DO. EUS-guided sampling of suspected GI stromal tumors. *Gastrointest Endosc.* 2009;69(7):1218-1223.
3. Philipper M, Hollerbach S, Gabbert HE, et al. Prospective comparison of endoscopic ultrasound-guided fine-needle aspiration and surgical histology in upper gastrointestinal submucosal tumors. *Endoscopy.* 2010;42(4):300-305.
4. Ponsaing LG, Kiss K, Loft A, et al. Diagnostic procedures for submucosal tumors in the gastrointestinal tract. *World J Gastroenterol.* 2007;13(24):3301-3310.
5. Demetri GD, von Mehren M, Antonescu CR, et al. NCCN Task Force report: update on the management of patients with gastrointestinal stromal tumors. *J Natl Compr Canc Netw.* 2010;8(Suppl 2):S1-S41; quiz, S42-S44.
6. Tran T, Davila JA, El-Serag HB. The epidemiology of malignant gastrointestinal stromal tumors: an analysis of 1,458 cases from 1992 to 2000. *Am J Gastroenterol.* 2005;100(1):162-168.
7. Dematteo RP, Gold JS, Saran L, et al. Tumor mitotic rate, size, and location independently predict recurrence after resection of primary gastrointestinal stromal tumor (GIST). *Cancer.* 2008;112(3):608-615.
8. Gold JS, Gonen M, Gutierrez A, et al. Development and validation of a prognostic nomogram for recurrence-free survival after complete surgical resection of localised primary gastrointestinal stromal tumour: a retrospective analysis. *Lancet Oncol.* 2009;10(11):1045-1052.

SECTION III

PANCREATIC

A 54-Year-Old Woman Has Weight Loss and Back Pain. An Ultrasound Is Suggestive of a Solid Mass in Her Pancreas. How Should Her Evaluation Best Proceed With Regards to Diagnosis and Staging?

Randall K. Pearson, MD

Pain and weight loss are the cardinal symptoms of pancreatic cancer (PC), but as these are nonspecific, the diagnosis is often delayed. In my referral practice, it is common for patients to undergo routine upper endoscopy, several months of empiric proton pump inhibitor therapy, and even the occasional laparoscopic cholecystectomy before appropriate cross-sectional imaging reveals the offending pancreatic mass. We have all been taught in medical school about the radiation of pancreatic pain into the back, most commonly precipitated by meals. In addition to pain, weight loss is at least equally due to the intense anorexia associated with PC. Glucose intolerance or overt diabetes precedes the diagnosis in the majority of patients and, if suspected in the appropriate patient (new-onset type 2 diabetes in a lean adult), might lead one to make an early diagnosis of PC.

In this brief scenario, the patient is not described as jaundiced so we can assume the lesion is in the body of the pancreas, given her pain. The pancreas is generally not well seen on transabdominal ultrasound. Our job is to establish the presence of a mass and accurately determine if the patient is a candidate for surgical resection by staging the presumed PC. However, tumor location and the presence of pain in this patient are poor prognostic indicators for an early-stage diagnosis; the pain usually reflects extension of

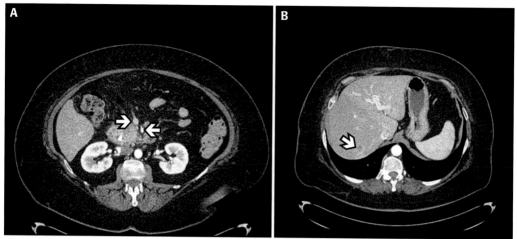

Figure 14-1. Arterial phase of a pancreas protocol dual-phase contrast-enhanced CT scan is shown in a patient presenting with abdominal pain, weight loss, and jaundice. (A) A low-density mass in the pancreatic head that is free of the superior mesenteric artery (upper arrow) and vein (lower arrow). (B) A low-density hepatic lesion later proven to be a metastasis is shown (arrow). This lesion was not seen on a routine CT performed elsewhere.

the disease along the mesentery, and pancreatic body lesions often grow large and metastasize before the primary symptom of pain develops.

A contrast-enhanced computed tomography (CECT) is the imaging test of choice at this point with a sensitivity of at least 90%. Magnetic resonance imaging (MRI) is less commonly performed in this setting but is an acceptable choice as well. For patients unable to undergo CECT, MRI has similar performance characteristics. A hypodense mass with contrast enhancement is consistent with ductal adenocarcinoma. Dual-phase imaging using contrast enhancement during the early arterial phase and later during the parenchymal perfusion ("pancreas protocol") is the single most accurate modality to establish the involvement of the mesenteric vasculature (implying stage III disease) or hepatic metastases (implying stage IV disease). For example, Figure 14-1A shows a typically hypodense lesion in the neck of the pancreas that is free of the mesenteric vessels. Figure 14-1B, from the same patient, shows a low-density hepatic lesion seen during the arterial phase that was not seen on a routine CECT done elsewhere, which was later proven to be a metastatic lesion. Figure 14-2 demonstrates the characteristic infiltration of the celiac artery, consistent with unresectable disease.

Unfortunately, we are faced with unresectable PC 80% to 85% of the time. For these patients, a biopsy to confirm the diagnosis is required, particularly if palliative chemotherapy or radiation is considered. For metastatic disease, a transabdominal ultrasound-guided biopsy of a liver metastasis is the most efficient diagnostic approach. If the disease is locally advanced, our practice is to proceed with an endoscopic ultrasound (EUS)-directed fine-needle aspiration (FNA) of the primary lesion along with concomitant celiac plexus neurolysis, especially if the pain is already requiring narcotics for control. At our center, in patients with resectable PC with a characteristic mass on CECT, a preoperative biopsy of the mass is not required to proceed with surgical resection, although many surgeons will not operate without a preoperative tissue diagnosis, and EUS-FNA in this setting is commonly performed.

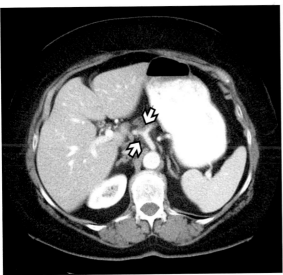

Figure 14-2. Unresectable PC. Tumor with the characteristic "cuffing" around the celiac artery is demonstrated and marked by the arrows. An EUS-directed FNA in this region confirmed the presence of adenocarcinoma infiltrating the perivascular space.

Virtually all patients with resectable PC have a mass in the pancreatic head and present with painless jaundice. The diagnostic and staging approach is the same as above. Endoscopic retrograde cholangiopancreatography (ERCP) is almost never required as a diagnostic test. A CT should always precede an ERCP to stage the disease and establish the goals of the ERCP. For example, if the CT shows unequivocal evidence of metastatic disease or locally extensive, unresectable tumor, a permanent self-expanding metal stent (SEMS) would be indicated for long-term palliation of biliary obstruction.

Furthermore, in our practice, if the PC is resectable and surgery is feasible within 7 to 10 days, we do not perform an ERCP preoperatively to decompress the biliary tree. Patients with obstructive jaundice rarely develop cholangitis unless instrumented. There is always the risk of causing post-ERCP pancreatitis that would either delay attempt at surgical resection or make an already high-risk surgery more difficult, although this is relatively unlikely to develop in patients with PC given the frequency of pre-existing pancreatic ductal obstruction and parenchymal atrophy. The counterargument has been that relieving jaundice preoperatively improves outcomes. This debate was the subject of a recently published multicenter randomized controlled trial from the Netherlands comparing preoperative endoscopic stenting followed by surgery versus immediate surgery.[1] Length of hospital stay, surgical complications, and mortality were not different between groups. Overall complications were higher in the preoperative biliary drainage cohort due largely to episodes of pancreatitis and cholangitis related to the ERCP or biliary stent. Unfortunately, this study had an exceptionally high level of ERCP-related cannulation failures and complications, and it is unclear if the results of this study can be generalized to routine clinical practice.

At least 30% of patients sent for surgical resection are found to have advanced disease at exploration, often due to small peritoneal or liver metastases. The role of further EUS staging in PC determined resectable by CECT is not clearly established. We perform EUS in patients with suspicion for more advanced disease in the following settings:

- High CA 19-9 levels (> 1000 mg/dL)
- Suspicious but inconclusive vascular involvement on CECT
- Suspicion of lymphadenopathy outside the area of typical surgical resection

In addition, I would always perform an EUS if the primary mass is not visible on CECT or if the imaging and clinical presentation suggest the possibility of an inflammatory process, especially autoimmune pancreatitis.

EUS is clearly superior to CECT in identifying lymph node involvement; however, involved nodes in the field of the planned surgical resection would not deny a patient an attempt at surgical resection at our center. Further refinement on the role of EUS in staging PC will likely be forthcoming as imaging improves.

Conclusion

When PC is suspected, cross-sectional imaging with CECT or MRI should be the first-line diagnostic test. Patients with a typical mass that appears resectable should be referred to a center capable of pancreatic resection before other invasive diagnostic or therapeutic procedures are done. Patients of unclear surgical status or in those in whom a tissue diagnosis is required should undergo EUS with FNA, often with concomitant ERCP.

Reference

1. van der Gaag NA, Rauws EAJ, van Eijck CHJ, et al. Preoperative biliary drainage for cancer of the head of the pancreas. *N Engl J Med.* 2010;362(2):129-137.

DO PATIENTS WITH PANCREATIC CANCER AND JAUNDICE NEED TO HAVE AN ENDOSCOPIC RETROGRADE CHOLANGIOPANCREATOGRAPHY PREOPERATIVELY?

Todd H. Baron, MD

The question of whether or not patients with pancreatic cancer and jaundice need to have an endoscopic retrograde cholangiopancreatography (ERCP) preoperatively has long been debated. Surgery for pancreatic cancer can either be curative or palliative. Curative resection is undertaken when there appears to be a tumor that is amenable to complete resection. Palliative surgery is performed when the tumor appears unresectable and is used to relieve biliary and/or gastric outlet obstruction via biliary enteric anastomosis (biliary bypass) and gastrojejunal anastomosis (duodenal bypass), respectively.

When we discuss preoperative ERCP in a patient with pancreatic cancer, we are referring to the patient with a potentially resectable cancer of the head of the pancreas. The operation in question is a pancreaticoduodenectomy (also known as a Whipple operation).

So, before considering ERCP, you must first establish whether the patient is a candidate for a Whipple operation. Resectability refers not only to the tumor itself but also to the patient's operative status. That is, would the patient be able to tolerate a major abdominal surgery? If the answer is yes, then the next question becomes is the lesion anatomically resectable? You need to determine resectability with a complete staging evaluation. This includes a pancreatic protocol CT scan to determine if there is invasion of blood vessels or presence of liver metastases that would preclude curative resection. In addition, endoscopic ultrasound (EUS) or magnetic resonance imaging (MRI) may also be used to determine resectability.

Now, why would you even consider sending your patient for an ERCP before attempted Whipple operation? The answer is that nearly all patients with cancer of the pancreatic head have bile duct obstruction and jaundice. This is because the bile duct courses through the head of the pancreas and becomes encased and/or compressed by tumor. In the early days of the Whipple operation, patients with deep jaundice did not seem to do as well postoperatively as those without jaundice. This may have been due to a variety of

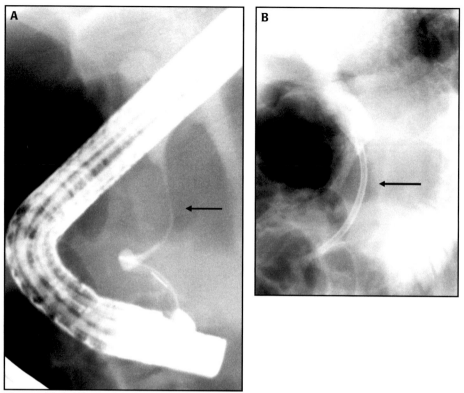

Figure 15-1. (A) Cholangiogram obtained during ERCP of a distal common bile duct stricture in a patient with pancreatic cancer in the head of the gland. (B) Fluoroscopic image obtained during ERCP demonstrating a plastic biliary stent placed across the stricture in the same patient (arrow).

factors. Nonetheless, when they became available, nonsurgical approaches were undertaken to relieve jaundice prior to surgery. This was initially achieved percutaneously and subsequently using ERCP. ERCP allows placement of a stent within the biliary tree across the stricture to relieve biliary obstruction (Figure 15-1). So, is this a good idea? The answer is yes and no. While in theory relief of obstructive jaundice with ERCP and stent placement could improve the outcome following Whipple resection, it cannot be done without the risks of complications associated with ERCP. These risks include sedation, infection (cholangitis), pancreatitis, perforation, and bleeding (if a biliary sphincterotomy is performed). The severity of these complications ranges from mild to severe, with most patients having no complications and most complications being mild in severity. Rare, severe complications not only require hospitalization (which could be prolonged) but may require surgery and even preclude the patient from ever having a Whipple operation. In addition, the technical success rate of ERCP with stent placement is not 100% and varies based mostly upon operator (endoscopist) experience. In centers with experienced endoscopists, the success rates of ERCP with stent insertion are high ($\geq$ 95%) with low complication rates ($\leq$ 5%).[1] So, in centers with expertise, the potential benefits often outweigh the risks. Historically, patients undergoing preoperative ERCP have received temporary plastic stents, which require maintenance via stent changes every 2 to 3 months. Newer,

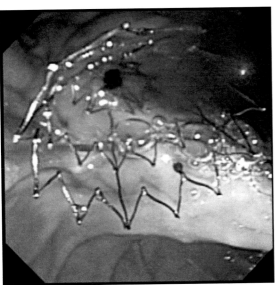

Figure 15-2. Endoscopic photo of an Alimaxx-B (Merit Medical Systems, Inc., South Jordan, Utah) uncovered metal biliary stent placed in a patient with pancreatic cancer undergoing neoadjuvant therapy prior to surgery. (Reprinted with permission of Douglas G. Adler, MD.)

expandable metal stents have been shown to provide prolonged patency when used for palliation of obstructive jaundice (Figure 15-2). There is a growing body of evidence that suggests that these stents are preferable in preoperative patients in whom surgery may be delayed more than 4 weeks.

Before we discuss which of your patients will benefit most from ERCP, we will look at the data on preoperative ERCP in pancreatic cancer patients. Detailed statistical analyses of published studies show that there is not convincing evidence that preoperative biliary placement either improves or worsens postoperative outcome, although it may cause more postoperative wound infections.[1] In addition, the pooled data show that preoperative biliary drainage prolongs hospital stay and increases cost.[2] Importantly, results from a recent randomized trial were published in which patients with cancer of the pancreatic head and obstructive jaundice underwent Whipple operation within 1 week of establishing resectability compared to those who underwent preoperative ERCP with stent placement followed by a waiting period of 4 to 6 weeks before undergoing Whipple operation.[3] In this last study, there was an initial ERCP procedural failure rate of 25%. In 46% of patients, there were ERCP-related complications; surgery-related complications were higher in the preoperative ERCP group without improvement in any outcome. This study may make you hesitant to ever ask for a preoperative ERCP again! However, it is important to realize that the complication rates from ERCP in this study were exceptionally high, certainly far higher than would be expected from most centers with expertise in ERCP and far higher than have been reported in other studies on preoperative ERCP. In addition, there are some patients who benefit from preoperative ERCP for relief of biliary obstruction. These include those jaundiced patients with acute cholangitis, those with pruritus, and those in whom any operation is likely to be delayed.[4] Delay in operating may be due to scheduling issues, need for preoperative evaluation and treatment of underlying comorbid medical illnesses, or because of administration of preoperative adjuvant (neoadjuvant) chemoradiation treatment. Neoadjuvant therapy is used routinely in many oncologic centers and delays surgery for 2 to 4 months.

So, do patients with pancreatic cancer and jaundice need to have an ERCP preoperatively? The answer is a definite maybe. First, it should not be performed routinely or solely for diagnostic purposes. You need to evaluate the patient's operative status and tumor resectability with a thorough medical evaluation and treatment of underlying comorbid medical illnesses using appropriate cross-sectional radiologic imaging studies and EUS. Then, you should consider whether preoperative oncologic treatment will be given. The selected patients listed above will very likely benefit from a preoperative ERCP when the procedure is performed by an experienced pancreaticobiliary endoscopist with a track record of high success and low ERCP complication rates.

References

1. Velanovich V, Kheibek T, Khan M. Relationship of postoperative complications from preoperative biliary stents after pancreaticoduodenectomy. A new cohort analysis and meta-analysis of modern studies. *J Pancreas.* 2009;10(1):24-29.
2. Wang Q, Gurusamy KS, Lin H, Xie X, Wang C. Preoperative biliary drainage for obstructive jaundice. *Cochrane Database.* 2008;(3):CD005444.
3. van der Gaag NA, Rauws EA, van Eijck CH, et al. Preoperative biliary drainage for cancer of the head of the pancreas. *N Engl J Med.* 2010;362(2):129-137.
4. Baron TH, Petersen BT, Mergener K, et al. Quality indicators for endoscopic retrograde cholangiopancreatography. *Gastrointest Endosc.* 2006;63(4 Suppl):S29-S34.

A 43-Year Old Woman Has Syncope Due to Hypoglycemia. An Insulinoma Is Suspected. Computed Tomography and Magnetic Resonance Imaging of Her Abdomen Are Negative. How Should This Patient Be Further Evaluated?

Sergey V. Kantsevoy, MD, PhD

Insulinomas are the most common hormone-secreting tumors, accounting for 60% of all pancreatic neuroendocrine tumors.[1] Patients with insulinomas usually present with clinical hypoglycemia, described by characteristic Whipple's triad of neurogenic (tremor, palpitation, anxiety, sweating, hunger, paresthesias) and neuroglycopenic symptoms (cognitive impairment, syncope, and behavioral changes often progressing to seizures and coma if untreated) associated with low blood glucose concentration. Most patients have prompt relief of all symptoms after the plasma glucose level is raised (by oral or intravenous administration of glucose).[2,3] The diagnosis of an insulinoma is confirmed by inappropriately high endogenous serum insulin concentration during a spontaneous or induced episode of hypoglycemia.[4]

Our clinical example of 43-year-old patient with symptomatic hypoglycemia and elevated serum insulin level raises a high suspicion of an insulinoma. Although the diagnosis of insulinoma is relatively straightforward in such a patient with clinically evident Whipple's triad and elevated endogenous insulin levels, the localization of the insulin-secreting tumor can be challenging because hormone-secreting neuroendocrine tumors are frequently very small at the time of the initial presentation (90% are less than 2 cm in size).[5] I usually start attempts of localization of suspected insulinoma with noninvasive tests (transabdominal

Figure 16-1. EUS image demonstrating insulinoma as a small (6 x 9 mm) hypoechoic rounded lesion located in the head of the pancreas.

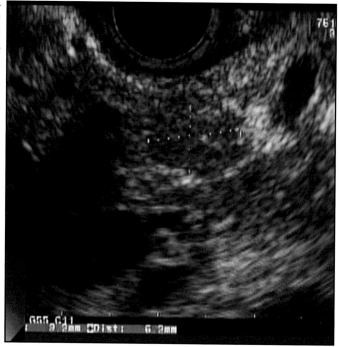

ultrasound, triple-phase pancreatic protocol CT, and/or MRI of the pancreas). However, these modalities are able to detect insulinomas only in 63% to 70% of the patients, leaving a significant minority without a clearly identifiable lesion.[6,7]

It is important to remember that in the proper clinical setting (patients with documented Whipple's triad), a negative imaging study does not exclude insulinoma.[8] If noninvasive imaging modalities fail to localize suspected insulinoma, I proceed with endoscopic ultrasound (EUS), which allows the generation of high-resolution images of the entire pancreas to search for an insulinoma.[1]

Using EUS, neuroendocrine tumors are visualized as oval-shaped or rounded lesions of various sizes inside the pancreas (Figure 16-1). Insulinomas can be hypoechoic (appearing darker and less echogenic than surrounding tissue), isoechoic (same echogenicity as surrounding tissue), or hyperechoic (which appear brighter than surrounding pancreatic tissue).[9] Isoechoic insulinomas cannot be visually differentiated from normal pancreatic tissue and are easily missed during EUS.[9] EUS alone can readily distinguish fluid-filled (cystic) and solid pancreatic lesions but cannot differentiate various types of solid tumors from each other by imaging alone.

To increase the diagnostic abilities of EUS, dedicated linear-array echoendoscopes were created. Linear array echoendoscopes allow EUS-guided sampling of the pancreatic lesions using a fine-needle aspiration (FNA) biopsy. However, the results of FNA should be interpreted with caution; a positive result (ie, presence of neuroendocrine or malignant cells) confirms the tissue diagnosis. At the same time, a negative result (absence of characteristic cells in the biopsy material) can be false-negative due to a sampling error during FNA, as smaller lesions are less likely to provide adequate tissue for a diagnosis.

In patients with suspected neuroendocrine pancreatic tumors, EUS is far superior to noninvasive tests (transabdominal ultrasound, CT, and MRI of the abdomen) with a reported sensitivity of 82%, specificity of 95%, and overall accuracy of 93%.[10,11] If traditional imaging studies (transabdominal ultrasound, CT, MRI, EUS) fail to localize the suspected insulinoma, you will need to order more invasive tests (mesenteric angiography, selective arterial calcium stimulation test with hepatic venous sampling) or even arrange exploratory laparotomy with intraoperative localization techniques (palpation, intraoperative ultrasonography, etc) in an attempt to identify a lesion for resection.[1,4,8]

Overall, most insulinomas can be detected preoperatively, but small insulinomas can present a challenge, and often multiple and/or repeated imaging or endoscopic studies are required to definitively localize and diagnose the lesion.

References

1. Goldfinger SE. Localization of pancreatic endocrine tumors (islet-cell tumors). UpToDate Web site. http://www.utdol.com/online/content/topic.do?topicKey=gi_dis/36370&selectedTitle=3%7E34&source=search_result. Accessed March 1, 2011.
2. Cryer PE, Axelrod L, Grossman AB, et al; Endocrine Society. Evaluation and management of adult hypoglycemic disorders: an Endocrine Society Clinical Practice Guideline. *J Clin Endocrinol Metab.* 2009;94(3):709-728.
3. Whipple AO. The surgical therapy of hyperinsulinism. *J Int Chir.* 1938;3:237-276.
4. Service FJ. Insulinoma. UpToDate Web site. http://www.utdol.com/online/content/topic.do?topicKey=endotumr/3014&selectedTitle=2%7E34&source=search_result. Accessed March 1, 2011.
5. McLean A. Endoscopic ultrasound in the detection of pancreatic islet cell tumours. *Cancer Imaging.* 2004;4(2):84-91.
6. Placzkowski KA, Vella A, Thompson GB, et al. Secular trends in the presentation and management of functioning insulinoma at the Mayo Clinic, 1987-2007. *J Clin Endocrinol Metab.* 2009;94(4):1069-1073.
7. Chen X, Cai WY, Yang WP, Li HW. Pancreatic insulinomas: diagnosis and surgical treatment of 74 patients. *Hepatobiliary Pancreat Dis Int.* 2002;1(3):458-461.
8. Service FJ. Diagnostic approach to hypoglycemia in adults. UpToDate Web site. http://www.utdol.com/online/content/topic.do?topicKey=diabetes/5055&selectedTitle=1%7E34&source=search_result. Accessed March 1, 2011.
9. Kann PH, Ivan D, Pfutzner A, Forst T, Langer P, Schaefer S. Preoperative diagnosis of insulinoma: low body mass index, young age, and female gender are associated with negative imaging by endoscopic ultrasound. *Eur J Endocrinol.* 2007;157(2):209-213.
10. Rosch T, Lightdale CJ, Botet JF, et al. Localization of pancreatic endocrine tumors by endoscopic ultrasonography. *N Engl J Med.* 1992;326(26):1721-1726.
11. Anderson MA, Carpenter S, Thompson NW, Nostrant TT, Elta GH, Scheiman JM. Endoscopic ultrasound is highly accurate and directs management in patients with neuroendocrine tumors of the pancreas. *Am J Gastroenterol.* 2000;95(9):2271-2277.

HOW SHOULD A CYSTIC PANCREATIC LESION BE EVALUATED PRIOR TO TREATMENT? WHICH CYSTIC LESIONS IN THE PANCREAS REQUIRE RESECTION AND WHICH CAN BE FOLLOWED CONSERVATIVELY?

Randall K. Pearson, MD

The widespread use of cross-sectional imaging has led to the increased recognition and awareness of pancreatic cysts. It is becoming increasingly clear that these cysts are not rare; the incidence of cystic pancreatic lesions ranges from 20% in necropsy studies to 0.7% to 1% among patients undergoing computed tomography (CT) or magnetic resonance imaging (MRI). However, the broad differential diagnosis for these cysts ranges from completely benign to malignant lesions. This creates a serious dilemma for the practicing physician, especially in light of the significant risks associated with pancreatic surgery.

The first task for the clinician is to determine if the cyst is symptomatic or not. When the cross-sectional imaging was performed for indications clearly unrelated to the pancreas, then the cyst is incidental. The patient with functional abdominal symptoms can present a challenge, but it is generally straightforward to discount a small pancreatic cyst as a cause for chronic dyspepsia or nausea. Symptoms that can be more reliably attributed to pancreatic cysts include acute pancreatitis, postprandial abdominal pain with weight loss, and jaundice. Pancreatic resection should be considered for these cysts to relieve symptoms and because they may have a higher risk of malignancy, although in clinical practice the vast majority of cysts faced by the practitioner will be asymptomatic and incidental.

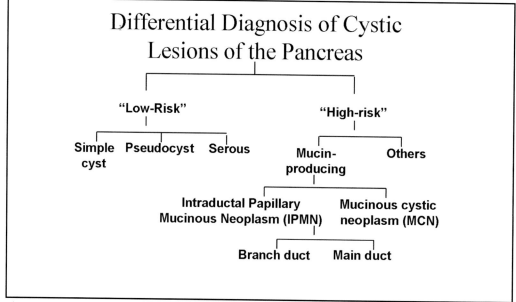

Figure 17-1. A diagnostic approach to pancreatic cysts based on risk of malignant transformation. The category "others" includes cystic degeneration of islet cell tumors.

A simple, but useful algorithm for the practical differential diagnosis used at our institution for pancreatic cysts is shown in Figure 17-1. In this approach, cysts are discriminated based on their risk for malignancy.

In older studies, pseudocysts were often listed as the most common pancreatic cysts, but this is no longer true in our practice. A clinical history of acute pancreatitis (especially if severe and if imaging demonstrates an evolution from acute fluid collection to walled off pseudocyst) or features of advanced chronic pancreatitis make the identification of pseudocysts relatively straightforward. Management is dictated by symptoms and development of complications.

Congenital or simple cysts are completely benign but are relatively uncommon in the pancreas. In my experience, they are generally small, and I do not recall our group sending patients with such lesions for pancreatic resection. A more common benign cyst is a serous cystadenoma, which is characterized by numerous, small, thin-walled cysts in a honeycomb pattern. Figure 17-2 shows the characteristic findings on CT imaging. These lesions can get quite large and will occasionally require resection because of a mass-like effect. The malignant risk is very low, and, if confidently identified, serous cystadenomas do not require surgery.

High-risk cysts are lined with mucin-secreting epithelium that is dysplastic. Mucinous cystic neoplasms (MCNs) are found almost exclusively in women and are generally a unilocular cyst in the body and tail of the gland. MCNs do not communicate with the pancreatic duct and can degenerate into an invasive cancer. Size is an important consideration; malignancy is rare in cysts smaller than 3 cm.

The most common neoplastic cyst is intraductal papillary mucinous neoplasm (IPMN). Affecting men and women equally, IPMN is characterized by a dysplastic, mucin-secreting epithelium that involves either the main pancreatic duct or its side branches, resulting in

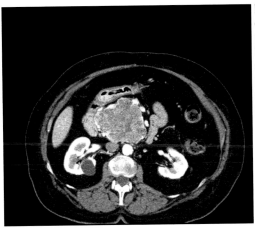

Figure 17-2. Serous cystadenoma. A large, well-encapsulated cystic mass is observed in the pancreatic head. Typical features include the honeycomb appearance of multiple small cysts enclosed in the larger lesion. Not shown is that, in spite of its size, there was no biliary or pancreatic duct enlargement consistent with a benign process.

duct dilatation and the formation of a cyst. When the main duct is involved, symptoms of acute pancreatitis, gland failure, "pancreatic" pain, and jaundice are common. Also, main duct IPMN is complicated by malignancy in up to 40% of patients. For these reasons, the management of main-duct IPMN is to proceed with surgical resection.

More commonly, IPMN involvement is restricted to the side branches (Br-IPMN). The risk of malignancy is low but the natural history and absolute risk of malignant transformation of these lesions is incompletely understood. Most are discovered incidentally, and many are small cysts in the head and uncinate process of the gland. The morbidity and mortality (at least 2% to 3%) of a Whipple resection gives the clinician pause in recommending surgical resection for these asymptomatic, low-risk lesions. One important caveat is the patient who presents with acute pancreatitis (often mild, self-limited) who is found to have a pancreatic cyst (typically in the uncinate process) that is inaccurately called a pseudocyst. Mucin secretion can cause main duct obstruction and secondary pancreatitis. Surgical resection is required to prevent recurrent attacks of pancreatitis.

Because the prevalence of overt malignancy in Br-IPMN is low (0% to 5%) and the annual development of cancer is no greater than 1% to 2%, consensus guidelines have been published based on the cumulative published experience with this condition.[1-3] At our center, we generally follow these guidelines in determining which patients are referred for surgical consultation versus imaging surveillance. Small cysts (less than 1 cm) can be followed with annual imaging; in my experience, very few of these lesions ever reach the threshold for resection.

The decision to watch cysts 1 to 3 cm in size is based on low-risk criteria of the cyst. Unfortunately, with the exception of the characteristic features of a serous cystadenoma, CT or MRI is unlikely to provide a confident diagnosis. Endoscopic ultrasound (EUS) provides additional imaging characteristics of the cyst wall and contents that predict a higher risk of malignancy including mural nodules and irregularity or thickening of the cyst wall. Further, the ability to perform fine-needle aspiration (FNA) allows for analysis of the cyst contents, including cytology and cyst fluid chemistries.

Surgical resection is recommended for cysts larger than 3 cm, but in practice, if a Whipple resection is needed, our surgeons have more confidence that the cyst is mucinous and poses a risk of malignancy in the asymptomatic patient. In centers with expertise,

EUS with FNA of the cyst is commonly used to enhance the diagnostic accuracy. While a positive cytology exam is very specific, in the published experience, the sensitivity for either diagnosing malignancy or a mucinous lesion is no greater than 50%. The single-best biochemical test on cyst fluid is CEA. High levels indicate with increasing confidence a mucinous lesion: more than 200 ng/mL is 80% specific and more than 800 ng/mL is virtually diagnostic of a mucinous lesion. Unfortunately, the level of CEA does not predict overt malignancy.

At the other extreme, very low CEA values are unlikely in premalignant mucinous lesions. If enough fluid is obtained, then measuring CA 19-9 can add some diagnostic confidence, because low CEA and CA 19-9 cyst levels are rarely seen in mucinous cysts. Cyst fluid CA 19-9 levels are very nonspecific and noninformative. Unfortunately, many cyst CEA levels fall between these extremes and are not particularly helpful in establishing a cyst as mucinous with accuracy rates hovering around 50%.

The following is a summary of my approach to the incidental pancreatic cyst.

- All decisions regarding resection have to take into consideration the patient's fitness for pancreatic surgery.

- Small cysts less than 2 cm can be followed with MR or CT surveillance at 6 months and then annually thereafter. New attention to radiation exposure risk makes MR an attractive modality.

- Location of the cyst is important; a body/tail lesion of 3 cm would more likely proceed directly to surgery without attempting to confirm it as mucinous when compared to a pancreatic head lesion requiring a Whipple resection. This is especially true for younger patients who are facing potentially decades of imaging surveillance.

- Most symptomatic cysts are due to either large cysts causing a local mass effect or main duct IPMN and warrant immediate surgical consultation.

- Virtually all cysts larger than 2 cm are investigated with EUS for high-risk features and cyst puncture for CEA determination.

- CEA levels help determine if a cyst is mucinous but do not identify malignant cysts.

- EUS can be very helpful in establishing a serous cystadenoma when CT/MR features are lacking. The finding of microcystic changes coupled with low CEA is reassuring to initiate a surveillance strategy.

- ERCP is rarely used for diagnostic purposes in IPMN.

- There are no guidelines and our group has no consensus on how long a stable, small cyst needs to be monitored. After 3 years, we will generally progressively increase the surveillance interval.

References

1. Khalid A, Brugge W. ACG practice guidelines for the diagnosis and management of neoplastic pancreatic cysts. *Am J Gastroenterol.* 2007;102(10):2339-2349.
2. Lahav M, Yakov M, Avidan B, Novis B, Bar-Neir S. Nonsurgical management of asymptomatic incidental pancreatic cysts. *Clin Gastroenterol Hepatol.* 2007;5(7):813-817.
3. Tanaka M, Chari S, Adsay V, et al. International consensus guidelines for management of intraductal papillary mucinous neoplasms and mucinous cystic neoplasms of the pancreas. *Pancreatology.* 2006;6(1-2):17-32.

WHAT IS THE ROLE OF METAL BILIARY STENTS IN PATIENTS WITH UNRESECTABLE PANCREATIC CANCER AND JAUNDICE?

Sergey V. Kantsevoy, MD, PhD

More than 33,000 people are diagnosed with pancreatic cancer in the United States every year.[1] Only 15% to 20% of the patients who are diagnosed with pancreatic cancer will have resectable disease at the time of initial presentation.[2] The median survival of these patients varies from 3 to 6 months (for patients with remote metastases) to 7 to 12 months (those with locally advanced, unresectable pancreatic cancer).[3] Patients with the cancer located in the pancreatic head usually present with obstructive jaundice and pruritis, and palliation of these symptoms and its consequences significantly improve patients' quality of life.

Endoscopic retrograde cholangiopancreatography (ERCP) has become the main therapeutic tool in palliation of biliary obstruction in patients with pancreatic cancer. If, prior to the ERCP, I am not sure whether the patient will be a candidate for surgical resection, I will place a plastic biliary stent of the largest available diameter (usually 10 Fr). If this patient will subsequently undergo surgical resection of the pancreatic cancer, the plastic stent can be easily removed prior to or, more commonly, during surgery.

In pancreatic cancer patients who are not surgical candidates (patients refusing or unable to tolerate surgery due to their general condition and those with locally advanced or metastatic disease), obstructive jaundice could be palliated with placement of either plastic or metal stents. Plastic stents are less expensive, but they are smaller in diameter (only 7 to 11.5 Fr) compared to metal stents, which expand to 10 mm (30 Fr) after placement. Due to a relatively small diameter, plastic stents rarely function longer than 2 to 3 months, and all will ultimately clog. If the patient's general condition is poor and his or her life expectancy is less than 3 months, I usually place a plastic stent, as the stent is likely to function until the patient's demise. However, my initial assessment of the patient's life expectancy could be wrong, and if this patient lives longer and then presents with an occluded plastic stent, it can always be exchanged for another plastic stent or changed to a metal stent.

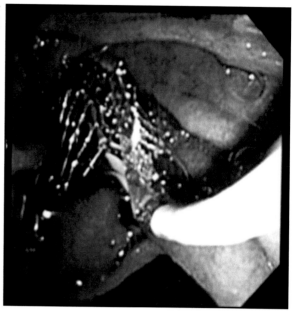

Figure 18-1. Proper position of the biliary metal stent through the major duodenal papilla in June 2009.

There are 2 major designs of self-expanding metal stents: uncovered (made of bare wire mesh) and covered (wire covered with a plastic coating). Stents may be partially covered or fully covered. The coating reduces tumor ingrowth through the stent and may increase the long-term patency of these devices compared to uncovered stents.[4,5] However, in patients with an intact gallbladder, a placement of a covered stent above the confluence between the cystic duct and common bile duct may block the cystic duct and can cause cholecystitis. To avoid such a complication, the proximal end of a covered biliary metal stent should be placed below the confluence with the cystic duct. If the patient's anatomy will not allow metal stent placement without blocking the entrance to the cystic duct, then an uncovered metal stent may be the best choice.

The length of the stent should be chosen to completely bypass the entire length of the occluded common bile duct and allow at least 5 to 10 mm of the stent above and below the occlusion. Deployment of the metal stent should be done under fluoroscopic and endoscopic observation. Fluoroscopic guidance allows precise control of the placement of the proximal end of the stent. At the same time, endoscopic observation allows us to control the position of the distal (intraduodenal) end of the stent in patients undergoing transpapillary stent placement. Appropriate position of both ends of the stent is equally important: if the proximal (biliary) end of the stent is too close to the site of the obstruction, it will be rapidly blocked by the tumor overgrowth. If the distal (duodenal) end of the stent is too short, it will be quickly blocked by the tumor ingrowth. If the distal end of the stent is too long, the stent can rub against the contralateral duodenal wall and cause erosions, ulcers, bleeding, and even perforation.

Properly placed metal biliary stents (Figure 18-1) usually last for at least 8 to 12 months.[6-8] However, the metal stents can be blocked by tumor ingrowth, sludge, and biliary stones (Figure 18-2). Patients with occluded biliary stents usually complain of skin itching, followed by dark discoloration of the urine and jaundice of the skin and sclera. The restoration of the biliary stent patency in patients with unresectable pancreatic

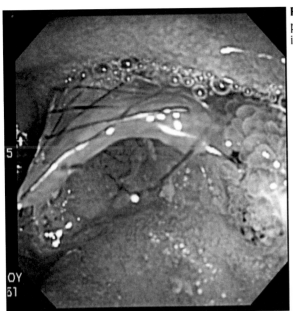

Figure 18-2. Tumor ingrowth caused complete occlusion of the biliary metal stent in April 2010.

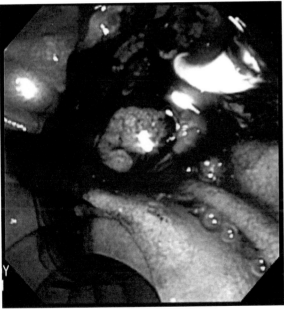

Figure 18-3. Extraction balloon pulled through the metal stent removing biliary sludge, stones, and debris.

cancer should be done as quickly as possible due to the risk of ascending cholangitis. Injection of contrast through the stent during ERCP confirms the level and extent of occlusion. Tumor, biliary sludge, stones, and debris can be removed by pulling the inflated balloon down through the occluded stent (Figures 18-3 and 18-4). Bleeding may occur but is usually self-limited. If stent occlusion is caused by tumor ingrowth through the wire mesh of the stent, the placement of a second metal stent inside the original stent can restore the luminal patency (Figure 18-5).

Figure 18-4. Metal stent patency restored.

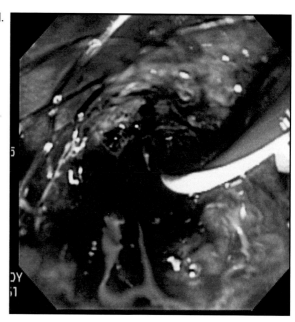

Figure 18-5. Second metal stent placed inside the originally placed biliary stent.

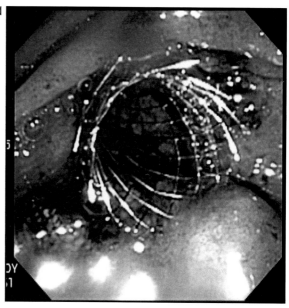

Overall, the decision of whether to place a metal or plastic stent should be individualized, and patients should be made aware of the relative risks and benefits of the options available.

References

1. Jemal A, Siegel R, Ward E, et al. Cancer statistics, 2006. *CA Cancer J Clin.* 2006;56(2):106-130.
2. Ryan DP, Mamon H. Management of locally advanced and borderline resectable exocrine pancreatic cancer. UpToDate Web site. http://www.utdol.com/online/content/topic.do?topicKey=gicancer/13604&selected Title= 28%7E29&source=search_result. Accessed March 1, 2011.
3. Fernandez-del Castillo C, Jimenez RE. Exocrine pancreatic cancer: palliation of symptoms. UpToDate Web site. http://www.utdol.com/online/content/topic.do?topicKey=gicancer/26915&selectedTitle= 2%7E29&source=search_result. Accessed March 1, 2011.
4. Isayama H, Komatsu Y, Tsujino T, et al. A prospective randomised study of "covered" versus "uncovered" diamond stents for the management of distal malignant biliary obstruction. *Gut.* 2004;53(5):729-734.
5. Krokidis M, Fanelli F, Orgera G, Rezzi M, Passariello R, Hatzidakis A. Percutaneous treatment of malignant jaundice due to extrahepatic cholangiocarcinoma: covered Viabil stent versus uncovered Wallstents. *Cardiovasc Intervent Radiol.* 2010;33(1):97-106.
6. Davids PH, Groen AK, Rauws EA, Tytgat GN, Huibregtse K. Randomised trial of self-expanding metal stents versus polyethylene stents for distal malignant biliary obstruction. *Lancet.* 1992;340(8834-8835):1488-1492.
7. Levy MJ, Baron TH, Gostout CJ, Petersen BT, Farnell MB. Palliation of malignant extrahepatic biliary obstruction with plastic versus expandable metal stents: an evidence-based approach. *Clin Gastroenterol Hepatol.* 2004;2(4):273-285.
8. Soderlund C, Linder S. Covered metal versus plastic stents for malignant common bile duct stenosis: a prospective, randomized, controlled trial. *Gastrointest Endosc.* 2006;63(7):986-995.

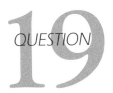

SHOULD PATIENTS WITH A STRONG FAMILY HISTORY OF PANCREATIC CANCER BE SCREENED FOR THE DISEASE, AND IF SO, HOW?

David Chu, MD and Douglas G. Adler, MD, FACG, AGAF, FASGE

The prognosis for pancreatic cancer (PC) continues to be poor (5%, 5-year survival rate). In 2009, PC will be the fourth highest cause of cancer-related deaths in the United States.[1] Most PC cases present as metastatic disease, with limited surgical and curative options. The overall 5-year survival rate with surgery remains around 20%.[2] The key to improved outcomes in PC is early detection of asymptomatic lesions. Currently, there are no established screening protocols for PC.

Pathophysiology of Pancreatic Cancer

Most PCs (80% to 90%) are adenocarcinomas that develop from epithelial cells in the pancreatic ducts or from resident stem cells. Precursor lesions, referred to as pancreatic intraepithelial neoplasias (PanIN), are classified as PanIN-1, PanIN-2, and PanIN-3 to reflect the amount of dysplasia present. A subset of PC develops from intraductal papillary mucinous neoplasms (IPMN), which, unlike PanINs, can be detected by conventional imaging (computed tomography [CT], magnetic resonance imaging [MRI], or endoscopic ultrasound [EUS]).

Risk Factors

PC is influenced by several risk factors. The most significant demographic factor is advancing age (80% of PCs occur between ages 60 and 80).[3] Male gender, Ashkenazi Jewish descent, and African-American descent are other demographic factors that mildly increase risk of PC.[4] Smoking and obesity are host factors that increase the risk of PC. Diabetes mellitus may be associated with increased risk of PC (OR of 1.82); however, the association is stronger with recently diagnosed diabetes (< 4 years) than long-standing diabetes (≥ 5 years).[5]

Family history of PC is a significant risk factor: 8% of patients diagnosed with PC have a first-degree relative with a history of PC.[6] Familial PC is a clinical syndrome that is associated with a moderate risk (< 10-fold) of developing PC and is defined as having 2 or more first-degree relatives with PC.

Certain genetic syndromes are associated with moderate to high risk of developing PC. Familial adenomatous polyposis (FAP), Lynch syndrome (hereditary nonpolyposis colorectal cancer), and hereditary breast/ovarian cancer (*BRCA1/BRCA2* gene mutations) are associated with a moderately increased risk (< 10-fold). Hereditary pancreatitis, Peutz-Jeghers syndrome, and hereditary melanoma due to *CDKN2A* gene mutations have been associated with the highest risk (> 10-fold).[4]

Challenges in Screening and Treating Pancreatic Cancer

The challenge in detecting PC at an early, treatable stage is that clinical symptoms are absent until most patients have achieved a significant tumor burden. There is a benefit in identifying early stage cancers (there is a 78% 4-year survival with stage I adenocarcinoma); however, these are rarely encountered in clinical practice.

Currently, there is no definitive screening protocol for PC. Efforts right now are focused on screening asymptomatic high-risk populations for developing PC.

High-Risk Groups

FAMILIAL PANCREATIC CANCER

As mentioned previously, familial pancreatic cancer (FPC) is defined by having at least 2 first-degree relatives affected with PC. The relationship between family size, number of family members affected, and exact relationship between family members is complex, and computer models are necessary to calculate the actual risk to the individual.[7] Early-onset PC (age < 40 years) in FPC kindreds was shown to have increased lifetime risk of developing PC (15.7% to 38.9%) as well.[8]

HEREDITARY PANCREATITIS

Hereditary pancreatitis is typically caused by mutations in the *PRSS1* gene (80%), which is associated with an increased risk for PC (up to 53-fold). The risk of developing PC is related to the duration and severity of pancreatitis attacks, as well as long-term endocrine failure (ie, diabetes).[9] Patient with *PRSS1* mutations who smoke tend to develop cancer 20 years prior to nonsmokers.

Cystic fibrosis (CF), which results from the inheritance of 2 mutated *CFTR* alleles, is associated with a significantly increased risk for PC. Inheritance of a single *CFTR* allele may confer a mild risk for PC.

SPINK1 and *CTRC* (chymotrypsin C enzyme) mutations are associated with increased risk of developing pancreatitis; however, the risk of developing PC is still undefined.

PEUTZ-JEGHERS SYNDROME

Peutz-Jeghers syndrome (PJS) is associated with a 132-fold increased risk in developing PC.[10]

HEREDITARY BREAST AND OVARIAN CANCER SYNDROME

Patients with hereditary breast and ovarian cancer syndrome have an increased risk of breast and/or ovarian cancers due to mutations in the *BRCA1* and *BRCA2* genes. *BRCA2* mutations are associated with a moderate risk (3.5- to 10-fold) of developing PC, whereas *BRCA1* mutations are associated with a mild risk (2-fold).[7] PALB2 gene mutations are also associated with PC. The PALB2 protein is a binding partner for BRCA2.

HEREDITARY MELANOMA DUE TO *CDKN2A* MUTATIONS

Approximately 10% of melanomas occur in family clusters, and *CDKN2A* gene mutations can be identified in approximately 40% of high-risk families.[11,12] Twenty-eight percent of *CDKN2A* families included at least 1 diagnosis of PC.

OTHER GENETIC SYNDROMES

Familial adenomatous polyposis (FAP) is caused by mutations in the *APC* gene and is strongly associated with developing colorectal cancer. FAP is associated with a low (4-fold) risk of developing PC.

Lynch syndrome is caused by mutations in any 1 of 4 mismatch repair genes (*MSH2, MLH1, MSH6,* or *PMS2*) and is associated with increased risk for developing colon, endometrial, and PCs.

Genetic Evaluation for Hereditary Pancreatic Cancer

The key to evaluating a patient for PC risk is to obtain a thorough family history that includes the types and ages of cancer diagnoses. Families that exhibit clusters of PC or other cancers (breast/ovarian, melanoma, etc) are candidates for genetic testing. In family members who present with cancer, genetic testing can be used as a tool to identify a specific mutation and appropriately offer genetic testing or increased surveillance for malignancy to at-risk relatives. For families without an identified genetic syndrome, tailored risk assessment can be provided based on empiric data.

Biomarkers in Screening: Serum-Based Markers

Currently, there are no effective screening biomarkers for PC. CA 19-9 has been the most studied (sensitivity 79%, specificity 82%); however, there are significant limitations.[13] Elevated CA 19-9 levels (to levels seen in malignancy) can be seen in benign processes (cholangitis, pancreatitis). Despite its weaknesses, no other biomarkers have been clinically proven superior to CA 19-9.

Screening With Imaging

No single imaging modality has been recognized as the gold standard for screening asymptomatic individuals for PC. CT, MRI/MRCP, and endoscopic ultrasonography (EUS) are the standard modalities, each of which has limitations. CT is relatively cheap, noninvasive, and readily available at most institutions. However, CT is insensitive for detecting small pancreatic lesions (< 15 mm) and is less sensitive than EUS in detecting PC.[14,15] There are also concerns regarding continuous radiation exposure in individuals who may be predisposed to cancer.

MRI with MRCP does not confer radiation exposure and has good sensitivity (84%) and specificity (97%) for detecting PC in the presence of ductal dilatation.[16]

EUS produces high-resolution images of the pancreas and can evaluate small focal lesions (2 to 3 mm). EUS was found to detect 49% more neoplastic lesions than CT or MRCP, independent of lesion size. EUS can be performed with fine-needle aspiration (FNA) to examine cytology of suspicious pancreatic lesions.

Initial Screening Attempts

Screening attempts for PC and precursor lesions have focused on high-risk populations. Imaging modalities used to screen included EUS/EUS-FNA, ERCP, and MRCP. Individuals with significant abnormalities on imaging were referred for exploratory surgery/resection. The results are summarized in Table 19-1.

Current Recommendations

The utility of PC screening remains controversial at this time. The overall dismal prognosis of PC and the lack of treatment options in advanced, metastatic disease suggest an urgent need to detect pancreatic malignancies when they are asymptomatic precursor lesions. However, screening the general population is not cost-effective, given the low incidence of PC, and there are no current data demonstrating improved survival from screening.

Screening studies of high-risk populations have found a high rate of pancreatic lesions (5% to 22%), suggesting that screening may be beneficial in selected groups.

Currently, individuals who are genetically predisposed for PC should be identified and referred to a multidisciplinary pancreatic team. They should be counseled about potential benefits and limitations of screening protocols and make their own informed decisions about pursuing screening. They should be educated regarding the clinical symptoms of PC as well as lifestyle factor modifications (smoking cessation, weight loss) to reduce further cancer risk factors.

<u>Table 19-1</u>

Results from Screening Studies for Pancreatic Cancer in Asymptomatic High-Risk Individuals

Study	High-Risk Population Studied	Imaging Modality	Total Yield
Brentnall et al[17]	FPC (14)	ERCP	0% (0/7)
Canto et al[18]	FPC (37), PJS (1)	EUS/EUS-FNA	5.3% (2/38): adenocarcinoma (1), IPMN (1)
Canto et al[19]	FPC (72), PJS (6)	EUS/EUS-FNA	10.2% (8/78): adenocarcinoma (1), IPMN (6), pancreatic endocrine neoplasm (1)
Poley et al[20]	FPC (21), PJS (2), *CDKN2A (13), HP (3), BRCA1 (3), BRCA2 (2), p53 mutation (1)*	EUS/EUS-FNA	22.7% (10/44): adenocarcinoma (3), IPMN (7)
Langer[21]	FPC and *CDKN2A* families (76)	EUS/EUS-FNA, MRCP	7.9% (6/76): PanIN (3), serous oligocystic adenomas (3)

References

1. Jemal A, Siegel R, Ward E, Hao Y, Xu J, Thun MJ. Cancer statistics, 2009. *CA Cancer J Clin.* 2009;59(4): 225-249.
2. Cameron JL, Riall TS, Coleman J, Belcher KA. One thousand consecutive pancreaticoduodenectomies. *Ann Surg.* 2006;244(1):10-15.
3. Lillemoe KD, Yeo CJ, Cameron JL. Pancreatic cancer: state of the art care. *CA Cancer J Clin.* 2000;50(4): 241-268.
4. Brand RE, Lerch MM, Rubinstein WS, et al. Advances in counseling and surveillance of patients at risk for pancreatic cancer. *Gut.* 2007;56(10):1460-1469.
5. Huxley R, Ansary-Moghaddam A, Berrington de Gonzales A, Barzi F, Woodward M. Type-II diabetes and pancreatic cancer: a meta-analysis of 36 studies. *Br J Cancer.* 2005;92(11):2076-2083.
6. Ghadirian P, Boyle P, Simard A, Baillargeon J, Maisonneuve P, Perret C. Reported family aggregation of pancreatic cancer within a population-based case-control study in the Francophone community in Montreal, Canada. *Int J Pancreatol.* 1991;10(3-4):183-196.
7. Shi C, Hruban RH, Klein AP. Familial pancreatic cancer. *Arch Pathol Lab Med.* 2009;133(3):365-374.
8. Brune KA, Lau B, Palmisano E, et al. Importance of age of onset in pancreatic cancer kindreds. *J Natl Cancer Inst.* 2010;102(2):119-126.
9. Lowenfels AB, Maisonneuve P, DiMagno EP, et al. Hereditary pancreatitis and the risk of pancreatic cancer. International Hereditary Pancreatitis Study Group. *J Natl Cancer Inst.* 1997;89(6):442-446.
10. Giardiello FM, Brensinger JD, Tersmette AC, et al. Very high risk of cancer in familial Peutz-Jeghers syndrome. *Gastroenterology.* 2000;119(6):1447-1453.

11. Florell SR, Boucher KM, Garibotti G, et al. Population-based analysis of prognostic factors and survival in familial melanoma. *J Clin Oncol.* 2005;23(28):7166-7177.
12. Goldstein AM, Chan M, Harland M, et al. High-risk melanoma susceptibility genes and pancreatic cancer, neural system tumors, and uveal melanoma across GenoMEL. *Cancer Res.* 2006;66(20):9818-9828.
13. Goonnetilleke KS, Siriwardena AK. Systematic review of carbohydrate antigen (CA 19-9) as a biochemical marker in the diagnosis of pancreatic cancer. *Eur J Surg Oncol.* 2007;33(3):266-270.
14. Legmann P, Vignaux O, Dousset B, et al. Pancreatic tumors: comparison of dual phase helical CT and endoscopic sonography. *AJR Am J Roentgenol.* 1998;170(5):1315-1322.
15. Tse F, Barkun JS, Romagnuolo J, Friedman G, Bornstein JD, Barkun AN. Nonoperative imaging techniques in suspected biliary tract obstruction. *HPB.* 2006;8(6):409-425.
16. Adamek HE, Albert J, Breer H, Weitz M, Schilling D, Riemann JF. Pancreatic cancer detection with magnetic resonance colangiopancreatography and endoscopic retrograde cholangiopancreatography: a prospective controlled study. *Lancet.* 2000;356(9225):190-193.
17. Brentnall TA, Bronner MP, Byrd DR, Haggitt RC, Kimmey MB. Early diagnosis and treatment of pancreatic dysplasia in patients with a family history of pancreatic cancer. *Ann Intern Med.* 1999;131(4):247-255.
18. Canto MI, Goggins M, Yeo CJ, et al. Screening for pancreatic neoplasia in high-risk individuals: an EUS-based approach. *Clin Gastroenterol Hepatol.* 2004;2(7):606-621.
19. Canto MI, Goggins M, Hruban RH, et al. Screening for early pancreatic neoplasia in high-risk individuals: a prospective controlled study. *Clin Gastroenterol Hepatol.* 2006;4(6):766-781.
20. Poley JW, Kluijt I, Gouma DJ, et al. The yield of first-time endoscopic ultrasonography in screening individuals at a high risk of developing pancreatic cancer [published online ahead of print June 2, 2009]. *Am J Gastroenterol.* doi:10.1038/ajg.2009.276.
21. Langer P, Kann PH, Volker F, et al. 5 Years of prospective screening of high risk individuals from familial pancreatic cancer families [published online ahead of print May 25, 2009]. *Gut.* doi:10.1136/gut.2008.171611.

A 78-Year-Old Woman With Pancreatic Cancer and Severe Pain Is Referred to You for Evaluation. What Is the Role of Celiac Plexus Neurolysis to Control Pain in These Patients?

Nikhil Banerjee, MD and Douglas G. Adler, MD, FACG, AGAF, FASGE

Pancreatic cancer is a commonly encountered gastrointestinal malignancy and is the fourth leading cause of cancer deaths in the United States annually. Pancreatic cancer typically affects patients 60 to 70 years old and presents with typical symptoms of epigastric abdominal pain, jaundice, and weight loss. Patients with pancreatic cancer often have a poor prognosis primarily because most present with advanced disease, thus ruling out potentially curative treatments such as surgery.

In many patients, pain associated with pancreatic cancer is a major focus of disease management. Pancreatic cancer pain is often severe and difficult to treat. Options for pain management include medications such as nonsteroidal anti-inflammatory drugs, acetaminophen, opioids, radiation therapy, chemotherapy, and celiac plexus neurolysis (CPN).

Celiac Plexus Neurolysis

The celiac plexus is a nerve ganglion located below the diaphragm in front of the diaphragmatic crura and anterior or next to the celiac artery. The celiac plexus contains a network of ganglia and interconnecting fibers primarily from the organs in the upper abdominal cavity, including fibers that transmit pain (nociception) from the pancreas.

CPN describes a technique in which alcohol or phenol, alone or in combination with a local anesthetic, is injected directly into, or in the vicinity of, the celiac ganglia, destroying visceral nociceptors in an attempt to lessen chronic abdominal pain. CPN is an alternative or additive tool in the management of pain due to pancreatic cancer and is widely employed in clinical cancer care.

Celiac plexus block (CPB) is another term that is often used interchangeably with CPN in the literature, although these terms refer to 2 distinct procedures with different indications and risks. CPB refers to the injection of a steroid and a local anesthetic into the celiac ganglia to provide temporary pain relief from chronic pancreatitis and will not be discussed further in this chapter.

Different techniques use different routes to reach the celiac plexus, different imaging modalities, and varying agents to perform the neurolysis. Surgery, computed tomography (CT)-guided injection, ultrasound, fluoroscopy, or endoscopic ultrasound can all be used as methods to administer these agents.

Surgical Neurolysis

CPN used to be performed through laparotomy or laparoscopy when unresectable disease is identified during surgery and is often performed in combination with palliative gastrojejunostomy and/or biliary bypass. The major advantage of this procedure is the ability to combine long-term palliation for all 3 primary symptoms of pancreatic cancer (pain, jaundice, and gastric outlet obstruction) in a single procedure. In the past, surgical treatment was the primary method for palliating these symptoms of pancreatic cancer. Improvements in initial tumor staging, a desire to avoid unnecessary surgery, and the rise of minimally invasive techniques such as radiology-based approaches or endoscopic ultrasound (EUS)-guided CPN have largely replaced surgery as a means of performing CPN.

Percutaneous Celiac Plexus Neurolysis

The celiac axis can be accessed percutaneously using a posterior or an anterior approach. This method of CPN is typically performed by anesthesiologists or interventional radiologists with radiologic guidance. Transcutaneous ultrasound or CT is typically used for radiologic guidance.

Endoscopic Ultrasound Neurolysis

EUS CPN, developed in 1996, has become more commonplace with better visualization of the celiac ganglia due to improvements in the technology used. The modern technique for endoscopic ultrasound-guided CPN uses a linear echoendoscope with Doppler. Transesophageal (in the very distal esophagus) or transgastric (in the very proximal stomach) are both standard approaches for this procedure. The needle is directed into the area of the celiac plexus, and a local anesthetic (typically bupivicaine) is injected, followed by a neurolytic agent (alcohol or phenol) (Figure 20-1). EUS-guided CPN appears to be as

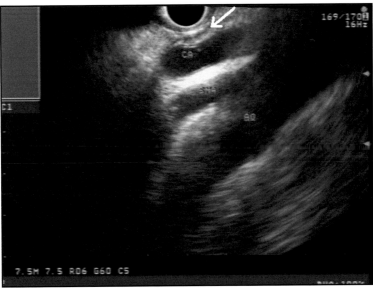

Figure 20-1. 7.5-MHz linear EUS image of the region of the celiac ganglia. The aorta (AO), celiac artery (CA), and superior mesenteric artery are all seen transgastrically. The needle for celiac neurolysis is typically passed through the gastric wall to the region just anterior to the origin of the CA where the ganglia is most commonly located. The arrow shows the intended needle path and destination.

effective and safe as other techniques, while being more cost effective because tumor staging via EUS-guided fine-needle aspiration (FNA) for tissue acquisition for a pathologic diagnosis and CPN can be performed all in one procedure.

Efficacy of Celiac Plexus Neurolysis for Pain Relief in Pancreatic Cancer

Several studies have examined the efficacy of CPN. These have largely demonstrated efficacy and subjective improvement in pain. Wong et al compared CPN via the posterior percutaneous approach to opioids alone in a double-blind randomized controlled trial. This trial demonstrated CPN (with opioids as needed) to be more efficacious in both decreasing pain intensity and improving quality of life when compared with opioids alone.[1]

Another study comparing both CPN and morphine treatment focused on both pain and quality of life in patients with pancreatic cancer pain. This study demonstrated that patients undergoing CPN had a significant increase in performance status with decreased pain.[2]

A recent systematic review examining the efficacy and safety of CPN compared with standard treatment in randomized controlled trials (RCTs) involving patients with unresectable pancreatic cancer further supported CPN as more effective than medication-mediated pain control.[3]

Intraneuronal injections have been evaluated in a small retrospective study at multiple-injection timepoints in patients with moderate to severe pain due to unresectable pancreatic carcinoma or chronic pancreatitis. Pain relief was reported in 94% and 80% of patients with pancreatic cancer and chronic pancreatitis respectively.[4] Intraneuronal injections have also been compared to perineuronal injections near or around the celiac plexus in a small cohort of patients with pancreatic cancer. Intraneuronal injection was felt to be as easy and safe to perform as perineuronal injection. This study did not see a difference in pain relief between injections into the 2 different locations.[5]

Safety and Complications of Celiac Plexus Neurolysis

Complications associated with CPN tend to be minor and commonly include local pain, diarrhea, and transient hypotension. A large meta-analysis of patients, the majority of which had pancreatic cancer, reported the following complications associated with percutaneous CPN: local pain (96%), diarrhea (44%), and hypotension (38%).[6] Serious neurological complications including lower extremity weakness and paresthesia, epidural anesthesia, and lumbar puncture occurred in 1% of patients. Significant non-neurologic complications occurred in an additional 1% and included pneumothorax, shoulder, chest and pleuritic pain, hiccoughing, and hematuria. The posterior approach was also associated with retroperitoneal fibrosis.[7] Other infrequent but serious complications, such as gastroparesis and gastric perforation, have been described in case reports.[8,9]

EUS- and CT-guided CPN have shown no serious complications reported with either technique. EUS has been shown to be preferred by patients who had experienced both procedures due to the lack of back pain and more sedation during EUS. In addition, EUS was found to be more cost-effective.[10]

Complications associated with EUS CPN have been reviewed in a clinical guideline published in 2005 by the American Society of Gastrointestinal Endoscopy (ASGE).[11] Perforation rate with EUS (for any indication) is less than 0.1% with no increase if FNA was performed. Infection risk ranges from 0% to 8%. The risk of pancreatitis is 0% to 2% in a pancreatic EUS-FNA. Mild intraluminal hemorrhage occurs in 1.3% to 4% of cases, and severe hemorrhage is infrequently reported.[12]

Risks specific to EUS with neurolysis include transient diarrhea (4% to 15%), orthostasis (1%), transiently increased pain (9%), and abscess formation, which is rarely reported.

Conclusion

Management of patients with pancreatic cancer is often directed toward palliation of symptoms with emphasis on pain control. Palliation of pain in pancreatic cancer often requires a multidisciplinary approach with options including oral analgesics, chemoradiation, and CPN.

CPN has long-lasting benefit in up to 70% to 90% of patients with pancreatic cancer regardless of the technique used. CPN is safe, with common, mild side effects and uncommon, severe adverse effects. CPN is a good alternative to opioid analgesics, both for improving pain control as well as avoiding or reducing the side effects of high-dose opioids. CPN does not appear to increase the lifespan in patients with pancreatic cancer.

CPN may be performed via endoscopic, percutaneous, or surgical routes. Although EUS-guided CPN is becoming more commonplace, there is currently no gold standard technique for performing CPN.

References

1. Wong GY, Schroeder DR, Carns PE, et al. Effect of neurolytic celiac plexus block on pain relief, quality of life, and survival in patients with unresectable pancreatic cancer: a randomized controlled trial. *JAMA.* 2004;291(9):1092-1099.
2. Kawamata M, Ishitani K, Ishikawa K, et al. Comparison between celiac plexus block and morphine treatment on quality of life in patients with pancreatic cancer pain. *Pain.* 1996;64(3):597-602.
3. Yan BM, Myers RP. Neurolytic celiac plexus block for pain control in unresectable pancreatic cancer. *Am J Gastroenterol.* 2007;102(2):430-438.
4. Levy MJ, Topazian MD, Wiersema MJ, et al. Initial evaluation of the efficacy and safety of endoscopic ultrasound-guided direct ganglia neurolysis and block. *Am J Gastroenterol.* 2008;103(1):98-103.
5. Adler DG, Hilden K, Thomas K, Wills J, Wong R. Endoscopic celiac plexus blockade via direct intraneuronal injection versus perineuronal injection: results of a pilot study [published ahead of print October 26, 2007]. *Am J Gastroenterol.* doi:10.1111/j.1572-0241.2007.01607.x.
6. Eisenberg E, Carr DB, Chalmers TC. Neurolytic celiac plexus block for treatment of cancer pain: a meta-analysis. *Anesth Analg.* 1995;80(2):290-295.
7. Michaels AJ, Draganov PV. Endoscopic ultrasonography guided celiac plexus neurolysis and celiac plexus block in the management of pain due to pancreatic cancer and chronic pancreatitis. *World J Gastroenterol.* 2007;13(26):3575-3580.
8. Takahashi M, Yoshida A, Ohara T, et al. Silent gastric perforation in a pancreatic cancer patient treated with neurolytic celiac plexus block. *J Anesth.* 2003;17(3):196-198.
9. Navarro-Martinez J, Montes A, Comps O, Sitges-Serra A. Retroperitoneal abscess after neurolytic celiac plexus block from the anterior approach. *Reg Anesth Pain Med.* 2003;28(6):528-530.
10. Gress F. A prospective randomized comparison of endoscopic ultrasound- and computed tomography-guided celiac plexus block for managing chronic pancreatitis pain. *Am J Gastroenterol.* 1999;94(4):900-905.
11. Adler DG, Jacobson BC, Davila RE, et al. ASGE guideline: complications of EUS. *Gastrointest Endosc.* 2005;61(1):8-12.
12. Gress F, Ciaccia D, Kiel J, Sherman S, Lehman G. Endoscopic ultrasound (EUS) guided celiac plexus block (CB) for management of pain due to chronic pancreatitis (CP): A large single center experience. *Gastrointest Endosc.* 1997;45:AB173.

A 70-Year-Old Man With Pancreatic and Liver Cancers Develops Gastric Outlet Obstruction Due to a Mass Compressing the Mass Proximal Duodenum. What Treatment Options Exist for This Situation?

Todd H. Baron, MD

Because the head of the pancreas lies adjacent to the medial wall of the duodenum, it is not surprising that, as cancer of the pancreatic head progressively enlarges, it often encases and/or extrinsically compresses the duodenum. This patient has malignant gastric outlet obstruction (GOO), a complication that almost always develops late in the course of pancreatic head cancer, often in the preterminal phase of the disease. Patients with GOO almost always have unresectable disease. Indeed, liver metastases are seen on computed tomography (CT) scan, and therefore the patient clearly has advanced incurable disease. Thus, any treatment approach is palliative, and the lifespan of the patient and underlying comorbid medical conditions need to be considered.

Traditional palliative treatment of malignant GOO is through surgical bypass. This is achieved using a loop gastrojejunostomy. In some centers, gastrojejunostomy is performed laparoscopically. However, many of these patients are debilitated and are poor operative candidates, particularly in the presence of malignant ascites. In addition, despite a good technical result, some patients have a poor functional result with continued nausea and vomiting after surgery.

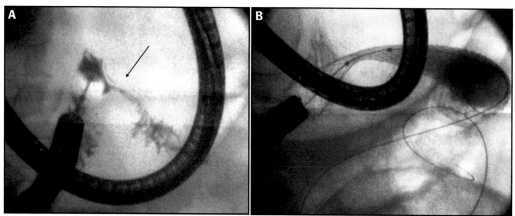

Figure 21-1. Fluoroscopic images of the placement of an expandable metal stent across a malignant duodenal stricture. (A) Duodenal stricture after contrast injection (arrow). (B) Same location following stent placement with contrast injection through the stent lumen.

A more recent option is placement of a self-expandable metal stent (SEMS) into the duodenum. This is a nonoperative procedure in which an endoscope is passed to the site of the lesion. Under fluoroscopic guidance, a guidewire is passed through the malignant stricture, and the stent, constrained in a sheath and mounted on a small (3-mm) delivery system, is passed over the guidewire through the endoscope channel and across the strictured bowel (Figure 21-1). The restraining sheath is then carefully withdrawn to allow the stent to deploy and expand with a resulting dramatic change in the luminal diameter of the stent and restoring patency of the bowel. Currently available fully deployed stents have a diameter of 22-mm in the midportion for an even greater lumen.

Gastroduodenal SEMS placement can be performed on an outpatient basis using moderate or deep sedation. Technical success rates (defined as proper stent placement across the lesion) are nearly 100% when performed by experienced endoscopists, and clinical success rates (defined as the ability to maintain hydration and nutritional status without enteral or parenteral supplementation) are approximately 90%. Some patients will fail to have clinical improvement despite a well-placed stent, likely due to diffuse gastroduodenal hypomotility or cancer-related anorexia, which can be very hard to treat and often requires jejunostomy feeding tubes and/or total parenteral nutrition (TPN). Gastric hypomotility is more commonly seen in gastric cancer as the stomach is likely to be infiltrated with tumor. Procedural complication rates of sedation, bleeding, and perforation are approximately 1%. Thus, endoscopic gastroduodenal SEMS placement is an attractive alternative to surgical bypass. However, delayed complications of SEMS placement can occur. The most common is stent occlusion with resultant recurrent symptoms of gastric outlet obstruction. Stent occlusion (up to 20%) occurs because the open mesh of the stent can permit tumor to grow between the openings (tumor ingrowth), from a benign tissue response to the metal (tissue hyperplasia), or from tumor outgrowing the ends of the stent (tumor overgrowth). Other less common complications include stent migration and delayed perforation, the latter of which often requires surgery. Stent occlusion generally can be managed by placement of another SEMS inside the original stent.

There have been many retrospective comparative studies of surgical gastrojejunostomy and endoscopic SEMS placement for palliation of malignant GOO. These studies show that SEMS placement provides rapid relief of obstruction with decreased cost and reduced hospital stays.[1] A recent small, randomized trial compared gastrojejunostomy (18 patients) and SEMS placement (21 patients) for palliation of malignant GOO.[2] The ability to eat improved more rapidly after stent placement (median 5 days compared to 8 days), but long-term relief was better after gastrojejunostomy. More major complications, more recurrent obstructive symptoms, and greater need for re-interventions occurred in the SEMS group. However, when stent obstruction was not considered as a major complication, no differences in complications were seen. No differences in median survival and quality of life were noted. The total costs of gastrojejunostomy were higher than SEMS placement, though not significantly. Based upon these results, gastrojejunostomy may be a better treatment option for good operative candidates with a life expectancy of more than 2 to 3 months, and SEMS may be the procedure of choice in those with more advanced disease and a poor performance status.

One important issue when SEMS are placed into the duodenum is the status of the biliary tree because patients who develop duodenal obstruction often have (or will have) biliary obstruction. This is most commonly seen in patients with pancreatic or ampullary cancer and is less commonly encountered in patients with, for example, gastric cancer. Placing a duodenal stent that crosses the region of the major papilla creates the possibility that future endoscopic access to the bile duct will be lost. This occurs because the papilla needs to be identified through the side of the duodenal stent, which is often difficult to do following stent placement. Thus, our approach is to perform endoscopic retrograde cholangiopancreatography (ERCP) with placement of an expandable metal biliary stent in all patients with known or impending biliary obstruction prior to insertion of the duodenal stent, if possible. We generally combine the ERCP with metal biliary SEMS placement and duodenal SEMS placement into one procedure to enhance efficiency. In the presence of obstructive jaundice and failed access to the bile duct because of duodenal obstruction itself or because of prior duodenal stent placement across the papilla, a percutaneous approach to the bile duct is usually performed for biliary stent placement.

Another less desirable option for palliation in this patient would be placement of a jejunal feeding tube with or without a gastric decompression tube. This would allow nutritional support without the need for parenteral supplementation and with relief of nausea and vomiting. This could be achieved percutaneously, endoscopically, or surgically. Disadvantages to this approach, which adversely affect quality of life, are that it does not allow the ability to resume peroral intake and requires external drains.

In the patient presented here, the presence of liver metastases suggests a limited survival time. You should consider an enteral stent placement with a concomitant biliary metal stent for this patient as the primary palliative treatment option. However, if expertise in laparoscopic surgery is available, then a palliative gastrojejunostomy would also be a good option.

References

1. Jeurnink SM, van Eijck CH, Steyerberg EW, Kuipers EJ, Siersema PD. Stent versus gastrojejunostomy for the palliation of gastric outlet obstruction: a systematic review. *BMC Gastroenterol.* 2007;7:18.
2. Jeurnink SM, Steyerberg EW, van Hooft JE, et al. Surgical gastrojejunostomy or endoscopic stent placement for the palliation of malignant gastric outlet obstruction (SUSTENT study): a multicenter randomized trial. *Gastrointest Endosc.* 2010;71(3):490-499.

A 67-Year-Old Man With Pancreatic Adenocarcinoma Undergoes Endoscopic Ultrasound, Which Reveals Malignant Adenopathy and Superior Mesenteric and Portal Vein Involvement. What Treatment Options Exist for This Patient?

Sean J. Mulvihill, MD

The treatment of pancreatic cancer is evolving with the development of new technologies and other advances in therapy. Despite these improvements, this tumor has the lowest 5-year survival rate of almost any other malignancy. Improved recognition of factors leading to elevated risk gives hope of surveillance, earlier diagnosis, and improved survival, although only a minority of affected patients fall into these groups and effective screening strategies are still under development. Diagnosis following the development of symptoms, especially painless jaundice as in this patient, remains the typical pattern. Atypical presentation modes, such as persistent vague abdominal pain, loss of appetite, unexplained weight loss, new-onset diabetes in a fit patient, and unexplained pancreatitis, should be recognized. Resection remains the only proven curative treatment. However, most patients present with advanced disease, either with metastases to distant organs or with locoregional disease that often precludes resection for cure, including some patients with vascular invasion and nodal metastases. At present, less than 20% of the 35,000 new cases diagnosed annually in the United States are candidates for surgical resection for cure.

Table 22-1

Cumulative Results of Published Single Institution Studies of Operative Mortality Following Whipple Resection

Papers Published	Average Operative Mortality (%)
1970 to 1979	18
1980 to 1989	7
1990 to 1999	2

Substantial improvements in operative mortality associated with resection have occurred during the past few decades (Table 22-1). However, these improvements have been more dramatic in centers of excellence with teams focused on the care of these patients than across the nation as a whole. These data suggest the need for quality improvement efforts in many hospitals across the nation or the referral of potentially resectable patients to centers with documented excellent perioperative results.[1,2]

Despite improvements in perioperative care and early outcome, long-term survival of patients with pancreatic adenocarcinoma remains poor. Of all patients, only about 4% can be expected to be living 5 years after diagnosis, and little improvement has been seen in the past 30 years. One of the major reasons for these poor results is the advanced stage at presentation of most patients at diagnosis and the relative lack of success of chemotherapy in substantially prolonging survival in patients with stage IV disease, despite numerous randomized controlled clinical trials testing novel approaches. In patients with resectable disease, 5-year survival rates range from 10% to 25% with median survival averaging about 18 months.[3] In the last 343 patients with pancreatic adenocarcinoma treated at the Huntsman Cancer Institute of the University of Utah, median survival in resected patients was 19.0 months but only 6.0 months in unresectable patients.

Nearly all reported series demonstrate an important negative impact of involved nodal status on survival. In our own experience following resection for pancreatic adenocarcinoma, median survival was 23 months in patients with N0 disease (absence of nodal metastases) and 16 months in patients with N1 disease (presence of nodal metastases). Twelve recent studies have analyzed the impact of portal vein or superior mesenteric vein invasion on survival.[3] Five of the 12 series report a significant negative impact of venous invasion on survival, but in 7 series, venous invasion did not significantly impact survival. Because of this, in recent versions of the AJCC staging of pancreatic cancer, venous invasion has been deleted as a factor in T staging. In our experience, and that of most reported series, vein resection has little negative impact on operative morbidity and mortality. Superior mesenteric artery and celiac artery invasion remain criteria for assigning T4 status and poorer prognosis. Most pancreatic surgeons also agree that the risk of resection rises substantially with arterial involvement. Most series demonstrate a significant impact of tumor size on survival, with lesions smaller than 2 cm having the best prognosis.[3]

In this patient, additional staging information is required to determine the possibility of resection for cure. National Comprehensive Cancer Network (NCCN) treatment guidelines suggest, at a minimum, chest imaging. Consideration should be given to positron-emission tomography (PET) staging and staging laparoscopy in patients such as this with possible nodal and/or venous involvement.[4] An assessment should be made regarding the suitability of the patient for major surgery. Review of patient factors, imaging, biopsy results, and treatment options in a prospective multidisciplinary treatment planning conference including experienced gastroenterologists, surgeons, medical oncologists, radiation oncologists, pathologists, and radiologists should occur. If the patient is unfit or unwilling to undergo potentially curative surgical therapy, endoscopic stenting to palliate biliary obstruction and jaundice and, if necessary, duodenal obstruction is the preferred approach.

For a fit patient such as this one who is willing to be treated with a 3-cm tumor, probable nodal involvement, and vein abutment, the choices are more complex. A critical decision is whether the surgeon believes the tumor to be "resectable," "borderline resectable," or "unresectable." Various centers use somewhat different criteria to define these categories. Emerging consensus, however, defines "resectable" as a tumor without distant metastases that can be removed with microscopically negative margins. The patient with vein abutment in this case usually would qualify as resectable, acknowledging that vein resection may be required. Patients with short segment vein encasement or hepatic arterial abutment are generally categorized as "borderline" resectable. Some patients with limited abutment of the inferior vena cava or left renal vein may also fit this category. Patients with more locally advanced tumors, including superior mesenteric arterial encasement, celiac arterial or aortic involvement, involvement of superior mesenteric vein branches in the small bowel or transverse colon mesentery, or distant metastases, are considered "unresectable."

In this patient, consideration should be given to factors of tumor size, probable nodal involvement, and venous abutment in selecting therapy. Either resection followed by postoperative adjuvant therapy or preoperative neoadjuvant therapy followed by resection followed by postoperative adjuvant therapy are acceptable options. No randomized studies comparing these strategies exist to demonstrate clear superiority of either approach. Consensus is emerging that surgery alone is inferior to surgery plus additional therapy, particularly chemotherapy, given in either a neoadjuvant or adjuvant fashion.

In our own center, we would favor a neoadjuvant approach, preferably in the context of a clinical trial, as no consensus on optimal combinations of chemotherapy agents or the role of radiotherapy exist. We would place an endoscopic stent in preparation for neoadjuvant therapy. Given the difficulties associated with plastic stent occlusion during chemoradiation, we prefer a metal stent, taking care to keep the proximal end above the tumor obstruction but below the cystic duct and certainly below the hepatic duct bifurcation to facilitate the creation of the surgical hepaticojejunostomy.

Tumor markers, particularly CA 19-9, and performance status are monitored during chemoradiation, and restaging with computed tomography is performed 4 weeks after completion of therapy. In this patient, if no radiographic progression is found and if performance status permits, resection is performed about 6 weeks after completion of neoadjuvant therapy. A rising CA 19-9 during treatment or declining performance status would usually lead to repeat PET/CT staging, looking carefully for signs of tumor progression precluding resection. In this situation, staging laparoscopy may also be advisable before committing to laparotomy. If resection is achieved, pathologic assessment of tumor response to therapy (eg, necrosis), nodal status, and margin status would help guide the decision for postoperative adjuvant therapy.

Unanswered questions in pancreatic cancer therapy include a poor understanding of the cell of origin and stimuli leading to the observed genetic changes in these malignancies. Resolution of competing hypotheses of the origin of pancreatic cancer in accumulated genetic insults in ductal epithelial cells, abnormal acinar to ductal cell metaplasia, and mutant stem cell precursors might dramatically alter therapeutic approaches in the future. Controversial clinical questions such as optimal neoadjuvant versus postoperative adjuvant therapy, optimal therapy for metastatic disease, and the role of regionalization of these complex patients remain unanswered today but are opportunities for clinical trials.

References

1. Teh SH, Diggs BS, Deveney CW, Sheppard BC. Patient and hospital characteristics on the variance of perioperative outcomes for pancreatic resection in the United States: a plea for outcome-based and not volume-based referral guidelines. *Arch Surg.* 2009;144(8):713-721.
2. Glasgow RE, Jackson HH, Neumayer L, et al. Pancreatic resection in Veterans Affairs and selected university medical centers: Results of the patient safety in surgery study. *J Am Coll Surg.* 2007;204(6):1252-1260.
3. Garcea G, Dennison AR, Pattenden CJ, Neal CP, Sutton CD, Berry DP. Survival following curative resection for pancreatic ductal adenocarcinoma. A systematic review of the literature. *J Pancreas.* 2008;9(2):99-132.
4. National Comprehensive Cancer Network. NCCN Guidelines in the treatment of pancreatic adenocarcinoma. http://www.nccn.org/professionals/physician_gls/PDF/pancreatic.pdf. Accessed April 26, 2010.

A 68-Year-Old Man Develops Painless Jaundice. Endoscopic Retrograde Cholangiopancreatography Demonstrates a Large Ampullary Mass. Biopsies Demonstrate Adenocarcinoma. How Should This Patient Be Managed?

Shyam J. Thakkar, MD and Douglas Pleskow, MD, AGAF, FASGE

Ampullary and pancreatic cancers originate in close proximity, but they are distinctly different disorders. The ampulla of Vater is a complex junctional structure uniting the common bile duct and ventral pancreatic duct to the duodenal lumen. It is often referred to as the major papilla and encompasses the sphincter of Oddi, the muscle complex encircling the distal portion of these ducts and a shared common channel. Ampullary cancer originates within this complex structure and, as a result, may have an intestinal or pancreatico-biliary histology depending on the site of origin (papillary or intra-ampullary [Figure 23-1]).[1] Ampullary carcinoma should not be confused with peri-ampullary cancers, which may arise from the distal common bile duct, pancreas, or adjacent duodenal mucosa. In advanced stages, peri-ampullary cancers may have overgrown the ampulla, making their site of origin difficult to determine.

The ampulla of Vater is the most common site of cancer originating in the small bowel. Additionally, the risk of ampullary cancer is increased by various polyposis syndromes, including familial adenomatous polyposis syndrome and hereditary nonpolyposis colorectal cancer. Despite these facts, ampullary cancer is a relatively rare malignancy, accounting for approximately 4 to 6 cases per million population and approximately 0.2% of all

Figure 23-1A. Diagram of sites of origin in ampullary cancer demonstrating papillary cancer arising from duodenal side of ampulla or cancer rising from the intra-ampullary portion of the papilla.

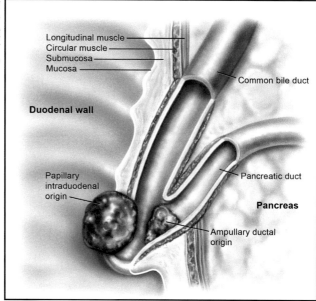

Figure 23-1B. Endoscopic photo of ampullary cancer visible from the duodenum.

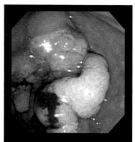

gastrointestinal tract malignacies.[2] A review of data from the National Cancer Institute's Surveillance, Epidemiology, and End Results (SEER) program found 5625 cases of ampullary cancer between 1973 and 2005; for unclear reasons, the frequency of the disease has been increasing since 1973.[3] In contrast, pancreas cancer is more common and is the fourth leading cause of cancer death in the United States. In 2009, approximately 42,470 new cases of pancreas cancer were diagnosed, and approximately 35,240 pancreatic cancer-related deaths occurred.[4] Although these disorders are often confused, ampullary and pancreatic cancers differ with regard to presentation, molecular characteristics, prognosis, and therapeutic options.

Clinical Presentation

Patients with ampullary cancer most commonly present with obstructive jaundice due to compression and/or obstruction of the distal bile duct by the tumor. Because of this anatomic origin, jaundice occurs early in ampullary carcinoma and generally when curative interventions are still attainable. Other presenting symptoms of ampullary cancer may include diarrhea due to fat malabsorption (steatorrhea), weight loss, and fatigue.

Up to one-third of patients with ampullary cancer may present with chronic, occult gastrointestinal blood loss with an associated microcytic anemia and/or heme-positive stools. An unusual but pathognomic sign of ampullary cancer is the passage of silver stool known as Thomas' sign (acholic stools mixed with blood will turn a silver color).[5]

Similar to ampullary cancer, pancreatic cancer may present with obstructive jaundice. However, this occurs if the tumor arises from the head of the pancreas and obstructs the intra-pancreatic portion of the common bile duct. Additionally, pancreas cancer may present with epigastric pain, weight loss, digestive problems, enlarged gallbladder (Courvoisier's sign), thrombo-embolic events, and diabetes. Although these symptoms lead to detailed evaluations, their presentation differs from that of ampullary cancer in that they usually occur at points when curative interventions are unattainable.

Prognosis and Molecular Characteristics

According to the American Cancer Society, the 1-year relative survival rate for all pancreatic cancer stages combined is 20%, and the 5-year relative survival rate is 4%.[4] These low rates are mainly due to the fact that, at the time of diagnosis, less than 10% of tumors are confined to the pancreas. The cancer has already spread, and in the major-ity of cases, it has progressed to the point where surgery is no longer a viable treatment option. In contrast, data show that patients with ampullary cancer have consistently better survival rates.[1,3,6-8] The obvious explanation for this difference is that ampullary cancers are detected relatively early due to the appearance of jaundice and thus have a more favor-able prognosis. There is also evidence to suggest that ampullary cancers are less aggres-sive than pancreatic cancers, which may be due to molecular differences between these cancers that favor better survival rates for ampullary cancer.[1,8] Data show that ampullary cancers, particularly intestinal type, have a lower incidence of epidermal growth factor receptor (EGFR) and mutant p53 over-expression and fewer activating K-ras mutations. This may contribute to the relatively favorable prognosis of ampullary cancer compared to pancreatic cancer, even in node-positive disease. Additionally, studies have shown that while p53 over-expression does occur in ampullary carcinomas, its presence is rare in precursor ampullary adenomas supporting a genetic alteration model of adenoma to carcinoma sequence similar to colorectal cancer as opposed to pancreatic cancer.[1,8]

Therapeutic Options

The surgical intervention for resectable ampullary cancers and certain pancreas can-cers (those arising from the head of the pancreas) is a pancreaticoduodenectomy (Whipple procedure). For premalignant ampullary adenomas, endoscopic or transduodenal resec-tion should be considered, and a Whipple procedure should be avoided if possible. The stag-ing of ampullary cancers is performed by the combination of computerized tomography (CT), endoscopic ultrasound (EUS), and endoscopic retrograde cholangiopancreatography (ERCP). These imaging modalities are also important in determining the endoscopic resectability of a premalignant ampullary adenoma. Ampullary carcinomas and advanced adenomas with ductal extension are better served with a Whipple procedure due to higher rates of incomplete resection and recurrence (Figures 23-2 and 23-3).[9] Endoscopic removal, in general, should not be attempted in patients with ampullary cancer.

Figure 23-2. EUS of an ampullary cancer with extension into the common bile duct. (Reprinted with permission of Manish Dhawan, MD, Western Pennsylvania Hospital.)

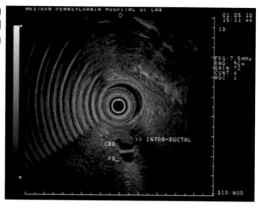

Figure 23-3. Cholangiogram showing intraductal extension of ampullary cancer manifesting as a distal filling defect in the common bile duct.

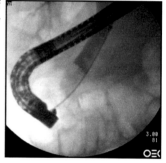

As with ampullary cancers, CT, EUS, and ERCP also play important roles in pancreas cancer. ERCP with metal biliary stenting can be therapeutic in patients with obstructive jaundice requiring neoadjuvant therapy or palliation. ERCP may also be diagnostic in cases where CT scan fails to reveal a pancreas mass and EUS is not available. Stenting of the injected duct should be performed at the time of ERCP in such circumstance. CT scan and EUS are complimentary technologies that allow for improved diagnostic accuracy and staging of pancreatic cancer. Such accuracy is essential in determining which patient would be best suited for surgical intervention with or without neoadjuvant therapy and those that should be treated palliatively.

In the current vignette of the 68-year-old man with painless jaundice, duodenoscopy with biopsy at the time of ERCP was diagnostic in determining the etiology of jaundice. Both a CT scan and EUS should be performed to accurately stage the ampullary cancer. If deemed resectable, curative resection in the form of a Whipple procedure should be attempted provided the patient is medically clear for the surgery. Depending on the stage, adjuvant chemotherapy may be necessary.

With regards to drainage, permanent, self-expanding metal stents should be placed in unresectable disease provided the biliary orifice can be identified and accessed. The role of preoperative biliary stenting in resectable ampullary cancer has not been widely studied. As such, preoperative endoscopically placed biliary stents may be dependent on several factors including surgical preference, whether patients are symptomatic with cholangitis or pruritis, or if a cholangiogram is performed at the time of ERCP.

Clinical Significance

While ampullary and pancreatic cancers are often associated and confused, there distinction as described is critically important as treatment is dependent on appropriate diagnosis and staging. Behavioral characteristics highlight the differences with improved outcomes in patients with ampullary cancer. However, with the introduction of neoadjuvant therapy coupled with surgery in high-volume centers, survival in pancreas cancer is being optimized.

References

1. Fisher WE, Bakey ME. Differences between ampullary, periampullary, and pancreatic cancer. *World J Surg.* 2007;31(1):144-146.
2. Behamiche AM, Jouve JL, Manfredi S, Prost P, Isambert N, Faivre J. Cancer of the ampulla of Vater: results of a 20 year population based study. *Eur J Gastroenterol Hepatol.* 2000;12(1):75-79.
3. Talamini MA, Moesinger RC, Pitt HA, et al. Adenocarcinoma of the ampulla of Vater: a 28-year experience. *Ann Surg.* 1997;225(5):590-600.
4. American Cancer Society. Pancreatic cancer. Available at http://www.cancer.org/Cancer/PancreaticCancer/DetailedGuide/index. Accessed April 2010.
5. Ogilvie H. Thomas's sign, or the silver stool in cancer of the ampulla of Vater. *Br Med J.* 1955;1(4907):208.
6. Berger HG, Treitschke F, Gansauge F, Harada N, Hiki N, Mattfeldt T. Tumor of the ampulla of Vater: experience with local or radical resection in 171 consecutively related patients. *Arch Surg.* 1999;134(5):526-532.
7. Roberts RH, Krige JE, Bornman PC, Terblanche J. Pancreaticoduodenectomy of ampullary carcinoma. *Am Surg.* 1999;65(11):1043-1048.
8. Takashima M, Ueki T, Nagai E, et al. Carcinoma of the ampulla of Vater associated with or without adenoma: A clinicopathologic analysis of 198 cases with reference to p53 and Ki-67 immunohistochemical expressions. *Mod Pathol.* 2000;13(12):1300-1307.
9. Lee SY, Jang KT, Lee KT, et al. Can endoscopic resection be applied for early stage ampulla of Vater cancer? *Gastrointest Endosc.* 2006;63(6):783-788.

SECTION IV

BILIARY

A 24-YEAR-OLD WOMAN IS FOUND TO HAVE PRIMARY SCLEROSING CHOLANGITIS. WHAT IS HER RISK OF DEVELOPING CHOLANGIOCARCINOMA?

James D. Morris, MD and Virendra Joshi, MD, AGAF

Primary sclerosing cholangitis (PSC) is a chronic, cholestatic liver disease marked by fibrosis and inflammation of the intrahepatic and extrahepatic bile ducts leading to biliary cirrhosis (Figure 24-1). Large proportions (60% to 80%) of patients have associated inflammatory bowel disease (IBD), most often ulcerative colitis. Cholangiocarcinoma (CCA) represents the most dreaded complication of PSC. CCA can occur at any location in the biliary tree and at any stage of PSC. The male-to-female ratio of CCA is 1.5:1, which parallels that of PSC patients overall.

The overall risk for the development of CCA ranges from a low of 7% in one natural history study to a high of more than 20% in patients referred for liver transplantation. CCA is rare in adults younger than 25 years of age but has been reported to occur even in teenagers. CCA generally develops in PSC patients in the 4th and 5th decades of life, usually in the absence of cirrhosis. It is important to recognize that 50% of patients with CCA are diagnosed within 1 year of diagnosis of PSC, suggesting that many patients may have subclinical disease for a protracted period of time. The incidence of CCA during follow-up starting 1 year after the diagnosis of PSC is 0.5% to 1.5% per year with no difference between males and females. The cumulative lifetime risk for developing CCA in PSC is around 20%.[1]

CCA in PSC most commonly presents as a stenotic perihilar lesion and occurs less commonly in the intrahepatic ducts or gallbladder. In PSC, distal bile duct tumors are rare (< 10%) and can sometimes be confused with pancreatic cancers involving the head of the gland. Histopathologically, infiltrating desmoplastic ductal type CCA is much more common than intraductal type. Often, in patients with PSC, a dominant stricture (defined as

Figure 24-1. Cholangiogram showing diffuse intrahepatic strictures in a patient with PSC.

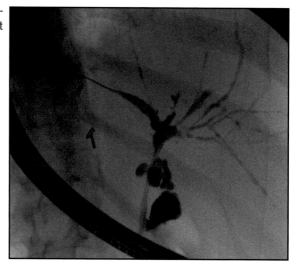

Figure 24-2. Cholangiogram demonstrating a tight distal common bile duct stricture in a patient with PSC that would be considered a dominant stricture (arrow).

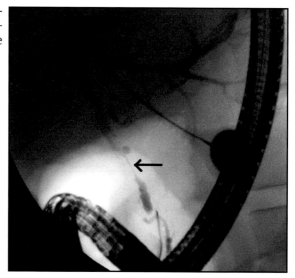

a stenosis with a diameter of less than or equal to 1.5 mm in the common bile duct or less than or equal to 1 mm in the common hepatic duct) is seen via cholangiography (Figure 24-2). Dominant strictures should be considered malignant until proven otherwise.

The risk factors for development of CCA in PSC are poorly defined. The proposed risk factors include duration of IBD, duration of PSC, and the presence of symptoms such as jaundice or weight loss. Alcohol use and smoking are also considered to increase the risk of malignancy in PSC. A yearly transabdominal ultrasound may be considered to screen for gallbladder cancer.

The diagnosis of CCA in the face of PSC, especially the ductal infiltrating desmoplastic type, is a challenge as the signs and symptoms of the tumor closely resemble the underlying disease (PSC). Clinically, malignancy should be suspected in patients with alarm features such as pruritus, jaundice, and weight loss.[2]

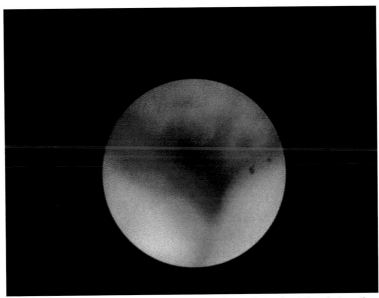

Figure 24-3. Cholangioscopy image of an intraductal, obstructing cholangiocarcinoma. Note the narrowed bile duct lumen.

Based on a study of 230 patients with complimentary imaging, the diagnostic value of carbohydrate antigen 19-9 (CA 19-9) level less than 20 U/mL as a serum marker has been noted to have a negative predictive value of 96% with an accuracy of 68% to exclude CCA. A value more than 129 U/mL has a positive predictive value of 100% and an accuracy of 90% to confirm CCA. However, in the presence of bacterial cholangitis, the CA 19-9 may be spuriously elevated; therefore, time for resolution of the infection must be allowed before consideration of the marker for risk assessment. Tissue markers like cytokeratin 7 and 19 have also been proposed but have not been validated in large number of patients. Brush cytology at the time of endoscopic retrograde cholangiopancreatography (ERCP) has very high specificity, but sensitivity is below 50%. The addition of fluorescent in situ hybridization (FISH) assays using DNA probes to look for cellular aneuploidy has improved sensitivity but cannot be viewed as a definitive testing modality in all patients.[3]

Radiographically, intrahepatic CCA in PSC may present as a mass lesion or an area of focal biliary dilation. Delayed "washout" of a suspicious lesion on a dynamic imaging study is suggestive of intrahepatic CCA. Perihilar CCA in PSC is more challenging as it is difficult to differentiate between benign and malignant strictures using standard imaging techniques. Indeed, 8% to 24% of hilar biliary strictures with suspected malignancy are ultimately found to be benign. Magnetic resonance imaging (MRI) with magnetic resonance cholangiopancreatography (MRCP) is a noninvasive and sensitive technique to visualize the biliary tree and the surrounding liver parenchyma. The combination of low serum tumor marker CA 19-9 (< 20 U/mL) along with 2 different imaging modalities showing negative results has high negative predictive value to exclude CCA. Interestingly, however, even in the presence of CA 19-9 more than 20 U/mL, abnormal findings on MRCP or ERCP, have positive predictive value of only 70%. Transpapillary cholangioscopy may be beneficial in the further evaluation of suspected strictures and can be used to diagnose malignancy using intraductal biopsies (Figure 24-3). Intraductal ultrasonography is another promising technique used to assess for malignancy in biliary strictures and is superior to endoscopic brush cytology. These techniques may only be available at tertiary centers specializing in the management of hepatobiliary disorders.

The presence of alarm features such as pruritis or jaundice in a patient with PSC should prompt evaluation of the hepatobiliary system. Initial evaluation is most appropriate with MRCP, which provides useful diagnostic information and can serve as a road map prior to any planned endoscopic intervention. ERCP in PSC imparts a risk of cholangitis and therefore should be reserved for patients with suboptimal imaging by MRCP or, more commonly, when tissue acquisition and/or therapeutic intervention is planned. When a dominant stricture is identified, ERCP-directed brush cytology and short-term biliary stent placement for duct decompression provide useful diagnostic and therapeutic value. If the endoscopic approach to bile duct decompression is unsuccessful, the patient may be referred for percutaneous biliary drainage. Prophylactic antibiotics should be given in all patients with PSC prior to any therapeutic procedure. Consideration should be given to surgical resection in noncirrhotic patients, and transplant referral should be made in the presence of cirrhosis. Prophylactic antibiotics are recommended in patients with recurrent cholangitis.[2]

Medical treatment with ursodeoxycholic acid in PSC has been shown to cause improvement in liver chemistries, but no improvement in survival. At this time, no treatment for PSC is available to prevent progression of disease and CCA.[4] Furthermore, treatment options for CCA in the background of PSC have been disappointing. Recent progress has been made with extended resection techniques and adjuvant radiochemotherapy prior to transplant with improved outcomes, but large scale data are still lacking, as many patients are incurable at the time of diagnosis. In the palliative setting, photodynamic treatment in conjunction with bile duct decompression with stent placement has also shown a survival advantage and improved quality of life. Without therapy, patients with CCA in the presence of PSC have a median survival of 5 months.

Conclusion

Young patients with PSC should be followed very closely for the development of alarm symptoms of CCA as these patients are at high-risk for developing CCA over their lifetime. Although no clear surveillance guidelines exist, the use of multiple modalities of imaging complemented by serial serum tumor markers and endoscopy may help to detect malignancy early.

References

1. Chapman R, Fevery J, Kalloo A, et al. Diagnosis and management of primary sclerosing cholangitis. *Hepatology.* 2010;51(2):660-678.
2. Watt KDS, Talwalkar JA, Wiesner RH. Primary sclerosing cholangitis and other cholangiopathies. In: Yamada T, ed. *Textbook of Gastroenterology.* 5th ed. Hoboken, NJ: Wiley-Blackwell; 2008:1978-2008.
3. Charatcharoenwitthaya P, Enders FB, Halling KC, et al. Utility of serum tumor markers, imaging, and biliary cytology for detecting cholangiocarcinoma in primary sclerosing cholangitis. *Hepatology.* 2008;48(4): 1106-1117.
4. Lindor K, Kowdley K, Luketic V, et al. High-dose ursodeoxycholic acid for the treatment of primary sclerosing cholangitis. *Hepatology.* 2009;50(3):808-814.

WHAT IS THE ROLE OF ENDOSCOPIC RETROGRADE CHOLANGIOPANCREATOGRAPHY AND ENDOSCOPIC ULTRASOUND IN PATIENTS WITH SUSPECTED CHOLANGIOCARCINOMA?

Rabi Kundu, MD, FRCS and Douglas Pleskow, MD, AGAF, FASGE

Malignant strictures of the bile duct due to cholangiocarcinoma are often difficult to diagnose and treat. These lesions generally present at an advanced stage due to a paucity of symptoms early in the disease.[1] Conventional imaging modalities such as transabdominal ultrasonography, computed tomography (CT), magnetic resonance cholangiopancreatography (MRCP), and positron emission tomography (PET) are often helpful investigations to provide information on the presence and extent of cholangiocarcinoma; however, the definitive diagnosis is generally dependent on obtaining tissue confirming malignancy from the biliary epithelium.

Endoscopic approaches represent the first-line approach to obtaining tissue from biliary strictures. The most commonly used endoscopic techniques for tissue acquisition include endoscopic retrograde cholangiopancreatography (ERCP) with cytology and endoscopic ultrasound (EUS) with fine-needle aspiration (FNA). Both of these are highly effective, but neither has a sensitivity and specificity for diagnosing cholangiocarcinoma that approaches 100%. Newer modalities have been tried to enhance the diagnosis of cholangiocarcinoma, which include digital image analysis (DIA), fluorescence in-situ hybridization (FISH), image-guided or cholangioscopic-aided biopsy, intraductal ultrasound (IDUS), cholangioscopy with narrow band imaging (NBI), and confocal laser endomicroscopy.

Endoscopic Retrograde Cholangiopancreatography

ERCP is the cornerstone of the diagnosis and management of cholangiocarcinoma. ERCP is excellent in delineating the anatomy of the entire biliary tree and for evaluating the presence and severity of any biliary strictures (Figure 25-1). Cholangiographic appearance

Figure 25-1. Occlusion cholangiogram of a patient with hilar cholangiocarcinoma. Note stricture at the common hepatic duct (arrow). (Reprinted with permission of Douglas G. Adler, MD.)

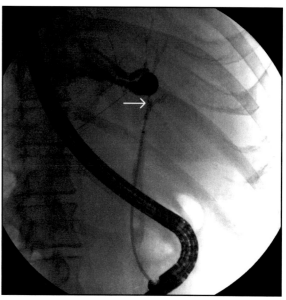

may, in general, suggest malignancy when a stricture is greater than 10 mm in length with irregular margins and demonstrates blunt margins, known as "shouldering."[2] A tissue diagnosis is required for definitive diagnosis of cholangiocarcinoma prior to treatment. Acquisition of tissue from the bile ducts during ERCP is obtained via brush cytology or biliary mucosal biopsy. ERCP and brush cytology has a specificity of approximately 100%; however, sensitivity is much lower, typically around 50% to 60%.[3-5] The low yield is most likely due to the hypocellular and desmoplastic nature of most cholangiocarcinomas. Dilation of a biliary stricture with a pneumatic balloon generally does not appreciably increase the yield of cytologic brushing.[3] In a study by deBellis, the diagnostic yield increased from 35% to 44% using this technique.[3] Performing a more aggressive dilation, our group demonstrated an increase yield of diagnosing cancer. Using an Howell Biliary Introducer Needle (HBIN; Wilson-Cook Medical, Winston-Salem, North Carolina) system the yield increased from 57% to 85%. The sequence of the technique was felt to be an important aspect in improving yield. A 10F HBIN introducer (Wilson-Cook Medical, Winston-Salem, North Carolina) was inserted through the biliary stricture. A biliary aspiration needle was then inserted into the stricture. A cytologic brush was then passed and tissue obtained. The conclusion was that these techniques disrupt the wall of the bile duct liberating malignant cells, thereby enhancing yield.[6] Comparing the cytology brush size (1.5 cm versus 5 cm) and bristles quality (soft versus rigid) did not increase the detection rates of malignant strictures.[7]

DIA has been evaluated due to the limited yield of brush cytology for the diagnosis for cholangiocarcinoma. DIA uses spectophotometric methods to quantify DNA content, chromatin distribution, and nuclear morphology. Aneuploidy or the presence of increased amounts of DNA suggests malignancy. DIA increased the sensitivity of brush cytology from 18% to 40%, but decreased the specificity from 98% to 77%.[8] Fluorescence in-situ hybridization uses a commercial probe to evaluate for polysomy of chromosomes 3, 7, 17, and 9p21. A sample is considered positive for malignancy if more than 5 cells show polysomy. Kipp and colleagues demonstrated that FISH increased brushing sensitivity from 15% to 34% and increased the specificity from 91% to 98%.[9]

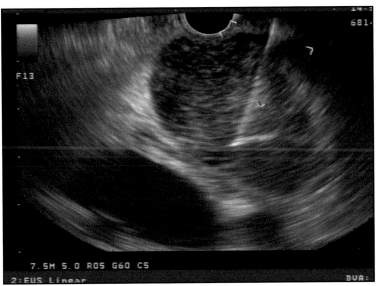

Figure 25-2. A 7.5-MHz EUS image demonstrating FNA of a 4-cm peri-portal lymph node in a patient with suspected cholangiocarcinoma. The portal vein is seen at the bottom left of the image. Cytologic analysis was positive for malignant cells, establishing the diagnosis. (Reprinted with permission of Douglas G. Adler, MD.)

Endoscopic Ultrasound-Guided Fine-Needle Aspiration Sampling

EUS with FNA is another technique used for diagnosing cholangiocarcinoma. CT-guided or ultrasound-guided biopsies often are not feasible because these tumors are usually small and isoechoic to the liver. These characteristics make them difficult to assess, especially when the tumor is located in the hilum. In patients with indeterminate biliary strictures after ERCP, EUS with FNA is very useful for evaluating these strictures and any surrounding lymph nodes. Although EUS can provide the data regarding the echotexture, size, shape, and borders of the stenosis and any associated mass, EUS images alone do not reliably differentiate malignant from benign lesions. EUS provides adequate visualization of the portal, hilar, celiac, and para-aortic lymph nodes. Tissue acquisition is imperative in establishing the diagnosis of cholangiocarcinoma. EUS-guided FNA of these lymph nodes is the most accurate modality to diagnose cholangiocarcinoma and helps with staging the disease (Figure 25-2).

The diagnostic sensitivity of EUS FNA ranges from 43% to 86% for all biliary strictures and 25% to 83% for proximal biliary strictures.[10-14] De Witt et al demonstrated the effectiveness of EUS FNA sampling of suspicious appearing biliary strictures following negative or unsuccessful ERCP. Seventeen of 24 patients with negative ERCP were found to have adenocarcinoma and 2 patients had confirmed benign disease. Five of the 24 patients had false-negative biopsies, confirmed at surgery (4 patients) and by survival of less than 2 months in one patient. The overall sensitivity was 77% with 100% specificity.[15]

Figure 25-3. Cholangioscopy image showing a malignant biliary stricture due to cholangiocarcinoma. (Reprinted with permission of Douglas G. Adler, MD.)

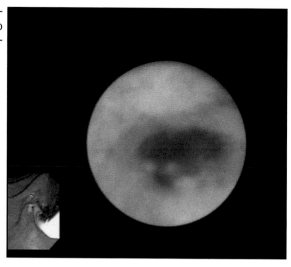

Figure 25-4. Cholangioscopy image of miniature forceps being used to directly biopsy a cholangiocarcinoma. (Reprinted with permission of Douglas G. Adler, MD.)

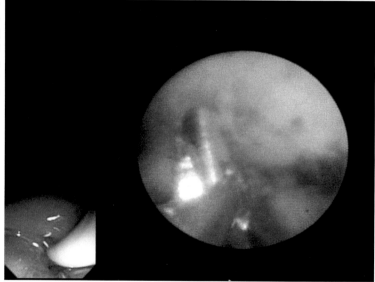

Other Modalities

ERCP with cholangioscopy with or without biopsy from strictures and filling defect has been shown to improve the sensitivity for the diagnosis for malignant lesions in the bile duct (Figures 25-3 and 25-4). In a study by Fukuda and his colleagues, all malignant lesions were diagnosed with this technique.[16] Shah and colleagues reported a sensitivity of 89% in their study with cholangioscopic-directed biopsy.[17] Tischendorf and his colleagues also demonstrated enhanced sensitivity of cholangioscopy with or without biopsy as compared to ERCP from 66% to 92%.[18] However this difference did not reach statistical significance in their study. Recently, Chen and Pleskow, using the Spyglass peroral cholangiopancreatoscopy system (Boston Scientific Corporation, Natick, Massachusetts) to obtain directed biopsies showed a sensitivity and specificity of 71% and 100%, respectively, in 27 indeterminate lesions.[19]

ERCP with intraductal ultrasound (IDUS) has a role in evaluating indeterminate bile duct strictures. It is also helpful in defining the longitudinal extent of the disease and as an adjunct for planning for surgery. Studies have shown effective increase in sensitivity in evaluating between benign and malignant strictures with ERCP and IDUS as compared to ERCP and tissue sampling. The ERCP with tissue sampling sensitivity ranged between 41% to 83% as compared with ERCP and IDUS 83% to 90% in these studies.[20-22] Compared to cholangiography, IDUS accurately defines the longitudinal spread of cholangiocarcinoma towards the liver (84% versus 47%) and towards duodenum (86% versus 43%).[23]

The emerging technology of narrow band imaging (NBI) and confocal laser microscopy show encouraging results in vivo. Meining et al examined 14 patients with biliary strictures.[9] Mucosal imaging was performed with a miniaturized confocal laser scanning miniprobe introduced via the accessory channel of a cholangioscope. Thereafter, targeted biopsy specimens were taken from the same regions. This technique had an accuracy rate of 86%, sensitivity of 83%, and specificity of 88% for diagnosis. The respective numbers for standard histopathology were 79%, 50%, and 100%. The mean signal-to-noise-ratio of laser microscopic images acquired from malignant strictures differed significantly from those of benign origin (1.8 versus 2.6; P = 0.005).[24] An international registry study is underway to validate this technology.

Conclusion

The definitive diagnosis of cholangiocarcinoma may be challenging. Initial evaluation with ERCP with tissue sampling is recommended. If the combination of ERCP, brush cytology, and biopsies are insufficient to provide a diagnosis, alternate techniques need to be considered. Cholangioscopy with directed biopsies has been demonstrated to be sensitive in diagnosing cholangiocarcinoma. EUS with FNA is effective in identifying and sampling lesions in and around the biliary tree. Newer modalities of evaluation including brush cytology with DIA and FISH hold great promise and are now becoming more available. IDUS can be used to evaluate biliary strictures prior to surgical resection if technology is available. NBI and confocal laser endomicroscopy for the evaluation of bile duct strictures represents a new technology that should be considered experimental at this time.

References

1. Lazaridis KN, Gores GJ. Cholangiocarcinoma. *Gastroenterology.* 2005;128(6):1655-1667.
2. Park MS, Kim TK, Kim KW, et al. Differentiation of extrahepatic bile duct cholangiocarcinoma from benign stricture at MRCP and ERCP. *Radiology.* 2004;233(1):234-240.
3. de Bellis M, Sherman S, Fogel EL, et al. Tissue sampling at ERCP in suspected malignant biliary strictures (part 2). *Gastrointest Endosc.* 2002;56(5):720-730.
4. Mansfield JC, Griffin SM, Wadhera V, Matthewson K. A prospective evaluation of cytology from biliary strictures. *Gut.* 1997;40(5):671-677.
5. Venu RP, Geenen JE, Kini M, et al. Endoscopic retrograde brush cytology. A new technique. *Gastroenterology.* 1990;99(5):1475-1479.
6. Farrell RJ, Jain AK, Brandwein SL, Wang H, Chuttani R, Pleskow DK. The combination of stricture dilation, endoscopic needle aspiration, and biliary brushings significantly improves diagnostic yield from malignant bile duct strictures. *Gastrointest Endosc.* 2001;54(5):587-594.
7. Fogel EL, deBellis M, McHenry L, et al. Effectiveness of a new long cytology brush in the evaluation of malignant biliary obstruction: a prospective study. *Gastrointest Endosc.* 2006;63(1):71-77.

8. Baron TH, Harewood GC, Rumalla A, et al. A prospective comparison of digital image analysis for the identification of malignancy in biliary tract strictures. *Clin Gastroenterol Hepatol.* 2004;2(3):214-219.

9. Kipp BR, Stadheim LM, Halling SA, et al. A comparison of routine cytology and fluorescence in situ hybridization for the detection of malignant bile duct strictures. *Am J Gastroenterol.* 2004;99(9):1675-1681.

10. Rösch T, Hofrichter K, Frimberger E, et al. ERCP or EUS for tissue diagnosis of biliary strictures? A prospective comparative study. *Gastrointest Endosc.* 2004;60(3):390-396.

11. Lee JH, Salem R, Aslanian H, Chacho M, Topazian M. Endoscopic ultrasound and fine-needle aspiration of unexplained bile duct strictures. *Am J Gastroenterol.* 2004;99(6):1069-1073.

12. Eloubeidi MA, Chen VK, Jhala NC, et al. Endoscopic ultrasound-guided fine needle aspiration biopsy of suspected cholangiocarcinoma. *Clin Gastroenterol Hepatol.* 2004;2(3):209-213.

13. Fritscher-Ravens A, Broering DC, Sriram PV, et al. EUS-guided fine-needle aspiration cytodiagnosis of hilar cholangiocarcinoma: a case series. *Gastrointest Endosc.* 2000;52(4):534-540.

14. Fritscher-Ravens A, Broering DC, Knoefel WT, et al. EUS-guided fine-needle aspiration of suspected hilar cholangiocarcinoma in potentially operable patients with negative brush cytology. *Am J Gastroenterol.* 2004; 99(1):45-51.

15. De Witt J, Misra VL, Le Blanc JK, McHenry L, Sherman S. EUS-guided FNA of proximal biliary strictures after negative or non diagnostic ERCP brush cytology results. *Gastrointest Endosc.* 2006;64(3):325-333.

16. Fukuda Y, Tsuyuguchi T, Sakai Y, Tsuchiya S, Saisyo H. Diagnostic utility of peroral cholangioscopy for various bile-duct lesions. *Gastrointest Endosc.* 2005;62(3):374-382.

17. Shah RJ, Langer DA, Antillon MR, Chen YK. Cholangioscopy and cholangioscopic forceps biopsy in patients with indeterminate pancreaticobiliary pathology. *Clin Gastroenterol Hepatol.* 2006;4(2):219-225.

18. Tischendorf JJ, Kruger M, Trautwein C, et al. Cholangioscopic characterization of dominant bile duct stenoses in patients with primary sclerosing cholangitis. *Endoscopy.* 2006;38(7):665-669.

19. Chen YK, Pleskow DK. Spyglass single-operator per oral cholangiopancreatoscopy system for the diagnosis and therapy of bile-duct disorders: a clinical feasibility study (with video). *Gastrointest Endosc.* 2007;65(6): 832-841.

20. Stravropoulos S, Larghi A, Verna E, Battezzati P, Stevens P. Intraductal ultrasound for the evaluation of patients with biliary strictures and no abdominal mass on computed tomography. *Endoscopy.* 2005;37(8):715-721.

21. Farrell RJ, Agarwal B, Brandwein SL, Underhill J, Chuttani R, Pleskow DK. Intraductal US is a useful adjunct to ERCP for distinguishing malignant from benign biliary strictures. *Gastrointest Endosc.* 2002;56(5):681-687.

22. Vazquez-Sequeiros E, Baron TH, Clain JE, et al. Evaluation of indeterminate bile duct strictures by intraductal US. *Gastrointest Endosc.* 2002;56(3):372-379.

23. Tamada K, Nagai H, Yasuda Y, et al. Transpapillary intraductal US prior to biliary drainage in the assessment of longitudinal spread of extrahepatic bile duct carcinoma. *Gastrointest Endosc.* 2001;53(3):300-307.

24. Meining A, Frimberger E, Becker V, et al. Detection of cholangiocarcinoma in vivo using miniprobe-based confocal fluorescence microscopy. *Clin Gastroenterol Hepatol.* 2008;6(9):1057-1060.

WHICH PATIENTS WITH CHOLANGIOCARCINOMA ARE CANDIDATES FOR SURGICAL RESECTION? IS LIVER TRANSPLANT AN OPTION FOR PATIENTS WITH CHOLANGIOCARCINOMA?

William R. Hutson, MD

Cholangiocarcinoma is an uncommon cancer and accounts for about 3% of all gastrointestinal malignancies and 10% of all primary liver cancers. The reported incidence is 1 to 2 cases per 100,000 population. Men and women are equally affected, and the majority of patients are older than 65 years. Cholangiocarcinoma is rarely associated with cirrhosis. Many patients with cholangiocarcinoma have no risk factors, but there are several conditions associated with an increased incidence. Those conditions are usually associated with proliferative changes or dysplasia of the bile duct epithelium. The most common of these is primary sclerosing cholangitis, and others include congenital hepatic fibrosis, Caroli's disease, choledochal cysts, infection with *Clonorchis sinensis* (most common cause in Southeast Asia), and biliary atresia.

Cholangiocarcinomas arise from the epithelial cells of the intrahepatic and extrahepatic bile ducts. Cholangiocarcinomas are most commonly located at the biliary confluence (50% to 60%). Distal bile duct tumors account for 20% to 30% of all cases. Intrahepatic tumors are seen in approximately 10% of all cases. There are 3 distinct macroscopic types of tumor: sclerosing, nodular, and papillary. Papillary tumors are more often resectable and have a more favorable prognosis than the nodular or sclerosing types. Longitudinal spread along the duct wall and periductal tissues is an important pathological feature of cholangiocarcinoma. Unfortunately, unlike hepatocellular carcinoma, effective screening does not exist for cholangiocarcinoma.

Figure 26-1. PET CT image of a hypermetabolic hilar cholangiocarcinoma (arrow). Note the presence of endoscopic stents in the biliary tree next to the tumor. (Reprinted with permission of Douglas G. Adler, MD.)

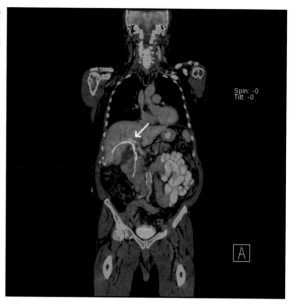

Radiographic studies are a mainstay in establishing the diagnosis of hilar cholangiocarcinoma and in selecting patients for surgical resection. While cross-sectional imaging may identify a hilar mass and proximal ductal dilatation, there often is no distinct mass visualized as these tumors are often isodense with the rest of the liver. Cholangiography is almost always required to identify the exact location of the tumor and the extent of biliary involvement. Magnetic resonance cholangiopancreatography (MRCP) has become a powerful investigative tool in these patients and can help serve to guide endoscopic and radiologic approaches to the bile ducts via endoscopic retrograde cholangiography (ERCP) and percutaneous transhepatic cholangiography (PTC) in many centers. Lastly, positron emission tomography used in conjunction with computed tomography scanning (PET-CT) has been used and may be very helpful for tumor localization, particularly for tumors greater than 1 cm in diameter and with a high rate of metabolic activity (Figure 26-1).

Serum levels of CA 19-9 are usually obtained when there is a suspicion for the diagnosis of cholangiocarcinoma but they are not sufficiently sensitive or specific for diagnostic purposes. The CA 19-9 may be elevated in benign conditions as well.

Surgical Options

Treatment of cholangiocarcinoma has remained challenging due to the lack of effective chemotherapy or radiation therapy and the aggressive nature of the disease. Partial hepatectomy is indicated for patients with anatomically resectable tumors who do not have cirrhosis. Partial hepatectomy is usually required to achieve the treatment goal of negative histologic margins and biliary-enteric continuity. Complete resection is the only treatment that offers the possibility of long-term survival in patients with intrahepatic cholangiocarcinoma. The 5-year actuarial survival of patients who have undergone curative resection is 17% with a median survival of 20 months.

Table 26-1

Contraindications for Resection in Patients With Cholangiocarcinoma

1. Presence of cirrhosis/portal hypertension.
2. Involvement of the main portal vein or hepatic artery by tumor.
3. Atrophy of one lobe with contralateral involvement of the portal vein branch or secondary biliary radicles.
4. Bilobar liver metastases.
5. Histologically proven N2 lymph node metastases.
6. Distant metastases.

Only a minority of patients with cholangiocarcinoma who are explored undergo resection (20% to 50%).[1] Many patients are unsuitable for resection, and criteria for unresectability are listed in Table 26-1. Most patients with unresectable disease die within 6 to 12 months of diagnosis.

The management of hilar cholangiocarcinoma has remained challenging due to the close proximity of key vascular and biliary structures, the lack of effective adjuvant therapy, and the difficulty of achieving complete resection due to the location and size of the tumor at the time of surgery. Resection of hilar cholangiocarcinoma involves complex surgery and generally requires an extended hepatectomy. The remaining liver remnant often consists only of segments 2 and 3, posing a risk for an inadequate remaining liver volume post-resection, which could result in a failure of regeneration of the remnant. In cases where the remaining liver volume is anticipated to be less than 25% to 30%, portal vein embolization of the same side of the tumor has been used to achieve hypertrophy of the future remnant prior to resection.

Distal cholangiocarcinomas, which can mimic pancreatic cancer with regards to presentation (painless jaundice with a distal common bile duct stricture), can be treated via pancreaticoduodenectomy (Whipple procedure). Patients with distal cholangiocarcinoma who do not meet criteria for resectability generally undergo palliative therapy that is aimed at relieving biliary obstruction and jaundice and preventing cholangitis.

Treatment of patients with hilar cholangiocarcinoma by liver transplantation has gained traction in recent years. Neoadjuvant chemoradiation in combination with liver transplantation for highly selected patients with hilar cholangiocarcinoma has shown impressive results with 5-year survival rates of approximately 76% to 82%. This is similar to other standard indications for liver transplantation, including hepatocellular carcinoma. The Mayo Clinic has performed and published data on the largest series of patients with hilar cholangiocarcinoma to have undergone liver transplantation.[2] Rigorous diagnostic criteria have been implemented to ensure the best outcome including tumor size less than 3 cm in radius, the findings of a malignant-appearing stricture confirmed by biopsy or cytology, an elevated CA 19-9 level more than 100 IU/mL, or evidence of aneuploidy in tissue samples. Unresectability is predicated based on technical considerations or the presence of intrinsic underlying liver disease. Exclusion of regional lymph node and peritoneal involvement is required by operative staging after completion of neoadjuvant therapy. Currently, there are only a handful of liver transplant centers performing this protocol in the United States, including the University of Utah. In certain United Network for Organ Sharing (UNOS) regions, patients are granted additional MELD points in order to accomplish transplantation more quickly as long as the protocol has been submitted and approved by the UNOS Liver and Intestinal Committee.[3]

Conclusion

Most patients with cholangiocarcinoma are not candidates for surgical resection due to advanced disease or poorly located disease. Partial hepatectomy, pancreaticoduodenectomy, and liver transplantation following neoadjuvant therapy are all viable options for carefully selected patients. These patients should receive treatment at high-volume centers to maximize results and minimize complications.

References

1. Petrowsky H, Hong JC. Current surgical management of hilar and intrahepatic cholangiocarcinoma: the role of resection and orthotopic liver transplantation. *Trans Proc.* 2009;41(10):4023-4035.
2. Rea DJ, Heimbach JK, Rosen CB, et al. Liver transplantation with neoadjuvant chemoradiation is more effective than resection for hilar cholangiocarcinoma. *Ann Surg.* 2005;242(3):451-458.
3. Schwartz JJ, Hutson WR, Gayowski TJ, Sorensen JB. Liver transplantation for cholangiocarcinoma. *Transplantation.* 2009;88(3):295-298.

WHAT ONCOLOGIC TREATMENT OPTIONS EXIST FOR PATIENTS WITH CHOLANGIOCARCINOMA WHO ARE NOT CONSIDERED SURGICAL CANDIDATES?

Kimberly Jones, MD

Patients with cholangiocarcinoma are, unfortunately, often diagnosed at an advanced stage, and, therefore, most are not candidates for potentially curative surgical therapy. Even with available therapy, these patients still have a short life expectancy of, on average, 6 to 12 months. The goal of treatment in patients who are not anatomically resectable or are not surgical candidates is palliation. As this disease usually affects patients in the seventh decade of life, comorbid conditions are important considerations in all aspects of treatment planning.[1] Because cholangiocarcinomas are rare and account for less than 3% of all gastrointestinal malignancies, there are limited data from randomized clinical trials to support most current oncologic treatments as standard of care, and further study is encouraged.[1] Furthermore, in the available studies on treatment, different subtypes of cholangiocarcinoma (which include intrahepatic, hilar, and extrahepatic lesions) were often combined with other pancreaticobiliary tumors (pancreas, gallbladder, and ampullary), making the data harder to interpret.

To determine resectability of a particular tumor, all clinical and radiological data should be reviewed at a multidisciplinary conference (Tumor Board) with the appropriate experts. If experts are not available locally, referral to a larger center should be made. Clinical staging is determined by one or more of the following: computed tomography (CT) scans, endoscopic retrograde cholangiopancreatography (ERCP), magnetic resonance imaging (MRI) with magnetic resonance cholangiopancreatography (MRCP), and/or and endoscopic ultrasound (EUS). Positron emission tomography (PET) scans can also be of value.

Still, despite the improvements in imaging modalities, up to 25% of patients thought to be resectable are found to have more advanced disease at exploratory laparotomy and are then deemed unresectable.[1] Cholangiocarcinoma is most commonly declared unresectable due to vascular invasion or due to significant involvement of the biliary tree, the presence of satellite or distant hepatic lesions, nodal involvement, and/or poor hepatic reserve. Retrospective reviews have shown that distal bile duct tumors are often more resectable than perihilar (Klatskin) tumors. Unfortunately, distal cholangiocarcinomas are rare. Stage III cholangiocarcinomas are generally unresectable and Stage IV are unresectable. Staging definitions are defined by the American Joint Committee on Cancer and updated regularly.

Patients with unresectable disease should undergo palliative biliary drainage by stent placement via ERCP or percutaneous drainage (a small percentage of patients will require both internal and external drainage to normalize their serum bilirubin). Patients can then be considered for a clinical trial if available, with options including chemotherapy and radiation, systemic chemotherapy alone, or best supportive care. A highly selected group of unresectable patients can be considered for liver transplantation after neoadjuvant chemotherapy and radiation. Neoadjuvant chemoradiation may allow for resection of a previously unresectable tumor. This is still an area in development, and this concept is currently being explored.

Data to support the optimal chemoradiation combination or systemic chemotherapy regimen for patients with advanced cholangiocarcinoma are lacking, and, therefore, participation in clinical trials is highly encouraged. The majority of published data comes from studies that include other hepatobiliary cancers and small numbers of patients in nonrandomized phase II trials. The use of radiation without chemotherapy has been controversial, with some data suggesting no overall survival benefit compared to historical controls and other data suggesting it improves pain and prolongs patency of the bile ducts and even overall survival.[2] These retrospective studies are hard to interpret given the varying types and doses of radiation and chemotherapy given. With the addition of concurrent chemotherapy using protracted infusional 5-fluorouracil (5-FU) and higher doses of radiation (with brachytherapy boosts), median survivals as high as 11.9 months have been reached.[2] More recently, an oral form of 5-FU, capecitabine, has been substituted for 5-FU in several chemotherapy regimens with apparent equivalency and is a reasonable option to combine with radiation. In general, combined chemoradiation should only be used in patients where all sites of disease can be captured within one radiation port. The newer techniques of delivering radiation, such as brachytherapy, stereotactic body radiotherapy (SBRT), and intraluminal radiation with yytrium-90 microspheres, deserve future attention and appear promising in localized disease.[1]

Even with local therapies such as chemoradiation, local spread along the ducts and into adjacent structures, as well as perineural invasion, is very common, and early perineural invasion is a poor prognostic factor for survival. Lymph node metastases usually involve hilar lymph nodes and, to a lesser extent, retroperitoneal lymph nodes and are also associated with a poor overall survival. Extrahepatic or hilar cholangiocarcinomas are more likely to have nodal involvement compared to intrahepatic tumors. Distant metastases are present in approximately 30% of patients at the time of diagnosis, and cholangiocarcinomas tend to spread into the peritoneal space, causing carcinomatosis and ascites, as well as spreading to the lung, bone, and distal lymph nodes. Once patients have metastatic disease, palliative chemotherapy alone is the best option along with best supportive care.

Until recently, there was no standard chemotherapy option recognized for patients with cholangiocarcinoma. In 2010, results from a large phase III trial (n = 410) were presented and showed a statistically significant improvement in overall survival with the addition of cisplatin to gemcitabine, compared to gemcitabine alone, with a median overall survival rate of 11.7 months compared to 8.1 months (p < 0.001). This trial (ABC-02) included all biliary tract tumors, but the majority of patients were diagnosed with cholangiocarcinomas (59%).[3] This trial also supported prior data from a number of small phase II trials that seemed to suggest that combination chemotherapy regimens improved survival over single-agent studies with either gemcitabine or 5-FU. Combinations of gemcitabine and capecitabine (an oral 5-FU analog) also appear promising, and a total of 4 phase II trials have demonstrated median overall survivals between 12.7 and 14 months.

Other combinations have also been tried with another platinum drug, oxaliplatin, with encouraging results and may be better tolerated by some than cisplatin.[4] Until another large phase III trial is completed, the standard regimen is considered to be gemcitabine with cisplatin, and future studies will likely build on this doublet with the addition of biological agents, such as antiangiogenic therapies or inhibitors of specific growth factor receptors or their pathways. Lastly, single-agent gemcitabine alone is very reasonable for patients with poorer performance status and for those not included in clinical trials as chemotherapy may improve their quality of life over best supportive care, at least for some period of time. Single-agent gemcitabine is also very well-tolerated in the majority of patients.

Best supportive care has historically been associated with a poor median survival of only 2 to 3 months, and oncological therapy using either chemotherapy or chemoradiation can be very palliative with regard to quality of life in addition to prolonging survival and should be considered for all patients. Further study of cholangiocarcinomas independently of other biliary tumors is needed to look for other trends in terms of response rate to different therapeutic agents as well as the newer biological or target agents. Biological differences between the different subtypes of cholangiocarcinomas (intrahepatic, perihilar, extrahepatic) may also help predict susceptibility to our therapies given the different pattern of growth, spread, and outcomes seen between them.

References

1. Aljiffry M, Walsh MJ, Molinari M. Advances in diagnosis, treatment and palliation of cholangiocarcinoma. *World J Gastroenterol.* 2009;15(34):420-426.
2. Shinohara ET, Mitra N, Mengye G, Metz JM. Radiotherapy is associated with improved survival in adjuvant and palliative treatment of extrahepatic cholangiocarcinomas. *Int J Rad Oncol Biol Phys.* 2009;74(4): 1191-2009.
3. Valle J, Wasan H, Palmer DH, et al. Cisplatin plus gemcitabine versus gemcitabine for biliary tract cancer. *N Engl J Med.* 2010;352(14):1273-1281.
4. Hezel AF, Zhu AX. Systemic therapy for biliary tract cancers. *Oncologist.* 2008;13(14):415-423.

SHOULD PATIENTS WITH UNRESECTABLE CHOLANGIOCARCINOMA AND JAUNDICE BE MANAGED VIA ENDOSCOPY WITH STENTS, INTERVENTIONAL RADIOLOGISTS WITH DRAINS, OR BOTH?

Allene Salcedo Burdette, MD

Cholangiocarcinoma is the second most common primary liver tumor, but overall it is rare. Its incidence, like that of hepatocellular carcinoma, is on the rise. Patients may be diagnosed with cholangiocarcinoma early if the common hepatic or common bile duct is involved. In these patients, biliary obstruction and jaundice will develop, and the patient will seek treatment earlier in the course of the disease. If the tumor is perihilar or intrahepatic, jaundice may not develop for some time, and the disease is more likely to be advanced at the time of diagnosis.

Making the diagnosis of cholangiocarcinoma can be challenging. Tissue is usually required for diagnosis and can be obtained percutaneously via needle or brush cytology, endoscopically with brushings or cholangioscopy-guided direct biopsy,[1] or via a transhepatic biliary approach with an atherectomy biopsy device.

As with hepatocellular carcinoma, surgical intervention provides the best chance for cure. Unfortunately, only a small percentage of patients are considered resectable at the time of presentation (Figure 28-1). Even with a complete surgical resection, recurrence rates can be as high as 50%, and metastatic rates can be up to 40%.

Other options for treating cholangiocarcinoma exist, including chemotherapy, radiation therapy, and photodynamic therapy. However, even with the use of such palliative measures, patients often require long-term drainage with either endoscopically placed stents or percutaneous biliary drainage (PBD) catheters placed by interventional radiologists (IRs).

Figure 28-1. Contrast-enhanced axial CT demonstrates a low attenuation cholangiocarcinoma centered in the right hepatic lobe, but extending to involve the medial segment of the left lobe. The mass causes central biliary obstruction, with bilateral biliary ductal dilatation.

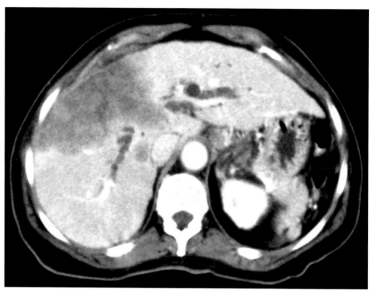

Deciding which method is best for drainage depends on several factors, including the patient's overall clinical status and local tumor anatomy. Percutaneous access is most appropriate when endoscopic management is not successful,[2] which is most commonly encountered in patients with Roux-en-Y anatomy in whom endoscopic retrograde cholangiopancreatography (ERCP) may not be technically possible.

When a patient is referred to me for PBD catheter placement, I make sure that an attempt has been made to stent endoscopically or that the patient has known postoperative anatomy that would obviate an endoscopic approach. If ERCP is technically feasible, it should be performed prior to attempts at PBD catheter placement.

Some patients have anatomy amenable to drainage by either means. The least invasive means of initial stent placement is endoscopic. While this method requires the use of sedation and, in some institutions, general anesthesia, it does not involve the traversal of hepatic parenchyma. If a plastic stent is placed, it must be exchanged for a new stent periodically, which typically occurs every 3 to 4 months. Exposure of the stent to bacterial microfilm, biliary sludge, and refluxed enteric contents results in occlusion of the stent over time, which can result in recurrent jaundice and possibly cholangitis. Endoscopic biliary stent placement is the most common palliative treatment for patients with malignant strictures and is considered the treatment of choice for hepatobiliary malignancies that are unresectable.[1,3]

A patient who undergoes placement of a percutaneous biliary drain by an IR usually does so for one of several reasons. Some patients may present with biliary sepsis and are sufficiently unstable that ERCP is unsafe. Other patients may have challenging anatomy, including postoperative anatomy with gastric bypass or Roux-en-Y reconstruction. Failure rates in the presence of such anatomy can be as high as 40%, although the ability to traverse postoperative anatomy and successfully perform ERCP in these patients is heavily dependent on local expertise.

Endoscopic management might also not be feasible depending on the location of the tumor. More distal tumors are frequently amenable to endoscopic stent placement.

Lesions higher in the biliary tree may not be accessible endoscopically and may require percutaneous treatment. Hilar lesions may be difficult to fully treat via endoscopy as there may not be adequate intraductal lumen for the placement of bilateral endoscopic stents.

Initial placement of a PBD catheter is more invasive and more painful than endoscopic stent placement because traversal of the hepatic parenchyma is required. The procedure is typically performed under conscious sedation with the use of midazolam and fentanyl. Success rates for placement of a PBD are greater than 93%.[4] An overnight admission may be necessary, depending on operator preference, to observe for complications. All subsequent exchanges of the PBD catheter are done on an outpatient basis under conscious sedation. Like plastic endoscopic stents, PBD catheters occlude and are usually exchanged every 3 to 4 months. PBD catheter occlusion generally results in recurrent jaundice and infection, most commonly sepsis and/or cholangitis.

Complication rates for PBD catheter placement are 0.5% to 2.5%. The most likely complications are hemorrhage and sepsis with rates of 2.5%.[4] Pain is frequently encountered following the placement of a new PBD catheter. Rarely, patients may develop renal failure from fluid losses via the PBD catheter.

If the patient's prognosis is poor and life expectancy is less than 6 months, a permanent metal biliary stent can be placed. The duration of the metal stent's patency should be longer than the patient's anticipated life expectancy. Placement of a metal stent improves quality of life by freeing the patient from routine exchange of PBD catheters or endoscopic stents.[1] Metal stents for nonoperative patients can be placed via endoscopic or percutaneous approaches once biliary access has been achieved. Use of the percutaneous approach should be considered if percutaneous access already exists, whether or not the biliary system is accessible endoscopically.

Under certain circumstances, patients whose initial attempt at endoscopic stent placement is unsuccessful may undergo placement of a PBD catheter. Once the PBD catheter is successfully internalized to the duodenum, the PBD catheter can be converted to an endoscopic stent. Using a rendezvous technique involving the endoscopist and the IR, a wire is passed through the PBD catheter from the external approach and is positioned in the small bowel. The wire is snared by the endoscopist, withdrawn through the endoscope, and used to insert the endoscopic stent.[1,5] A simpler version of this technique involved placement of an endoscopic stent next to an existing transampullary PBD catheter, with subsequent PBD catheter removal. A reverse technique can also be done if initial endoscopic access is successful, and there is need for a PBD catheter. The endoscopist performs an ERCP, and the IR uses the cholangiogram to obtain definitive percutaneous access. Alternatively, if an endoscopic wire can be inserted to where an external drain is in place, the wire can be snared percutaneously and used to internalize the PBD catheter (Figure 28-2).

Both endoscopic stents and PBD catheters are well-tolerated by patients. The major benefit of a PBD catheter is the ease of the routine exchange. Patients who have an internal-external PBD catheter, which crosses the site of the tumor and terminates in the small bowel, are able to have the catheter capped and drain their bile internally. This allows them to be rid of the cumbersome external drainage bag. Some patients are committed to external drainage because their ducts are isolated from central drainage. This usually occurs because the PBD catheter cannot be positioned across the site of stricture or obstruction (Figure 28-3).

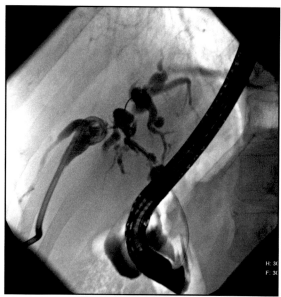

Figure 28-2. Cholangiogram demonstrates a rendezvous procedure with an external PBD looped in an inferior segment duct. An endoscope is in place with a wire extended, in an attempt to internalize the PBD.

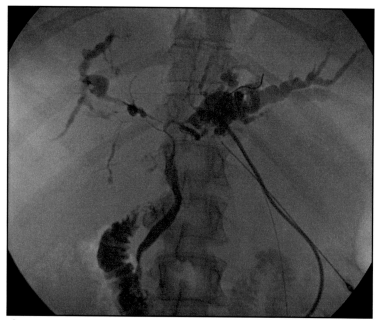

Figure 28-3. Cholangiogram from placement of a second external PBD demonstrates an existing external PBD, which has not been internalized to the duodenum due to the presence of Klatskin's tumor. This patient is a poor candidate for endoscopic drainage because of the peripheral involvement of disease.

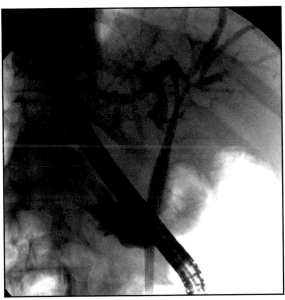

Figure 28-4. ERCP demonstrates bilateral plastic endoscopic stents placed to relieve biliary obstruction related to a Klatskin tumor. Central involvement by the tumor, with relative sparing of the distal ducts, makes this patient ideal for endoscopic management.

The major disadvantage of the PBD catheter is that the catheter extends outside the body. For some, it serves as a constant reminder of their diagnosis and all it entails. For others, it is inconvenient and may be a source of physical limitation. Another downside is the possibility of inadvertently dislodging the catheter. Even the most conscientious of patients may accidentally pull out or displace the PBD catheter while changing their clothes or getting out of a car. The inconvenience of having a drainage bag is better tolerated by some than others, and it is often difficult to predict who will tolerate external drainage well or poorly. Pain or skin site irritation is also an issue, as is the presence of an external foreign body, which places the patient at risk for infection.

The most obvious benefit of the endoscopic stent is that it is completely internal (Figure 28-4) and it is less likely to be dislodged. Infection is likely only in the face of stent occlusion. The stent's presence is known to none but the patient. An additional benefit is that internal drainage is more physiologic.

Some patients benefit from or require the placement of both percutaneous and endoscopic stents. This can be seen in patients with complex anatomy, incomplete biliary drainage via endoscopic approaches, or those undergoing neoadjuvant therapies for cholangiocarcinoma prior to liver transplantation. In this last situation, the PBD catheter can be used for treatment with brachytherapy (Figure 28-5).

With some exception, given the choice, most patients would elect to have an endoscopic stent, but either method of drainage is a viable option. It should be stressed that these are complementary techniques and that, in most institutions, gastrointestinal endoscopists and IRs work together closely on a daily basis to coordinate the care of patients with complex biliary disease. Anatomy usually dictates which approach is used, as well as the patient's overall clinical status. The availability of local expertise should also serve to guide therapy.[1,2]

Figure 28-5. Cholangiogram demonstrates a left endoscopic stent and right PBD. Originally, this patient had bilateral endoscopic stents but required percutaneous access for brachytherapy to treat a hilar cholangiocarcinoma.

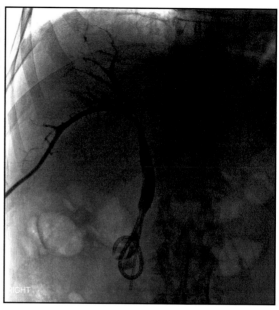

References

1. Singhal D, van Gulik T, Gouma D. Palliative management of hilar cholangiocarcinoma. *Surg Oncol.* 2005;14(2):59-74.
2. Kloek J, van der Gaag N, Aziz Y, et al. Endoscopic and percutaneous preoperative biliary drainage in patients with suspected hilar cholangiocarcinoma. *J Gastrointest Surg.* 2010;14(1):119-125.
3. Mallery J, Baron T, Dominitz J, et al. Complications of ERCP. *Gastrointest Endosc.* 2003;57(6):633-638.
4. Burke D, Lewis C, Cardella J, et al. Quality improvement guidelines for percutaneous transhepatic cholangiography and biliary drainage. *J Vasc Interv Radiol.* 2008;8(4):677-681.
5. Liu Y, Wang Z, Wang X, et al. Stent implantation through rendezvous technique of PTBD and ERCP: the treatment of obstructive jaundice. *J Dig Dis.* 2007;8(4):198-202.

WHAT IS THE ROLE OF PHOTODYNAMIC THERAPY AND BRACHYTHERAPY IN PATIENTS WITH CHOLANGIOCARCINOMA?

Ananya Das, MD, FACG, FASGE

Most cholangiocarcinomas (CCAs) are extrahepatic; approximately 60% to 70% are located in the hilar area (also known as Klatskin's tumors), and approximately 20% to 30% are located more distally, involving the common bile duct. Surgical treatment offers the only chance for cure for CCA, but only a minority of patients are surgical candidates. Even for these patients, an R0 resection is feasible in only about 30% of instances, and 5-year survival rates after R0 resection for hilar CCA are 10% to 40%, and for distal extrahepatic CCA are 25% to 40%. In patients with primary sclerosing cholangitis (PSC), which is by far is the most common risk factor for CCA, coexistent advanced liver disease, the possibility of multifocal cancer, the inherent risk of recurrent cholangitis with a biliary-enteric anastomosis, and their increased risk for further CCA makes the outlook of surgical therapy even more dismal.

Whenever you see a patient with CCA, you should recognize that relief of obstructive jaundice is a very important goal of therapy. Palliation of biliary obstruction, which reduces the morbidity associated with cholestasis and the risk of cholestatic liver failure, becomes a cornerstone of treatment of these patients. In my center, the majority of patients with CCA are candidates for endoscopic palliative treatment. Surgical palliative interventions such as debulking or biliary bypass are inferior to endoscopic palliation. Endoscopic stenting remains the most widely available and commonly used palliative treatment in these patients. In my practice, percutaneously placed external biliary drainage is usually reserved for patients in whom endoscopic stenting is not technically feasible, such as following gastric bypass surgery.

Photodynamic Therapy

Photodynamic therapy (PDT) has recently emerged as an attractive option for palliation of biliary obstruction caused by CCA. PDT requires intravenous administration of a photosensitizer, which is selectively retained by neoplastic tissue. The photosensitizer is usually a hematoporphyrin derivative (porfimer sodium). Light activation of the active drug is performed 40 to 96 hours after systemic administration of the photo-active drug via a quartz fiber mounted with a cylindrical diffuser tip coupled to a dye laser diode emitting a wavelength of 630 nm, with an energy density in the range of 180 to 240 J/cm^2. In the presence of the proper wavelength of light, the drug generates reactive oxygen species, which cause direct tissue damage. Light activation is performed in my center via transpapillary access during endoscopic retrograde cholangiopancreatography (ERCP), although this can also be performed via the percutaneous approach. The depth of tumor necrosis is about 4 to 6 mm. The other photochemical used for PDT is 5-aminolevulinic acid. This agent is less commonly used because it causes limited tumor necrosis to a depth of only 2 mm. Cutaneous photosensitivity is an inherent side effect of PDT and is reported in up to 25% of patients, with some patients developing significant injury.

PDT has become an important palliative modality for CCA based on its positive impact on survival, which has been reported in several case series and in 2 recent randomized controlled trials. In a randomized controlled trial in patients with unresectable CCA when compared to stenting only, PDT resulted in significant prolongation of survival (median: 493 days versus 98 days). It also improved biliary drainage and quality of life. Indeed, this study was terminated prematurely because PDT proved to be so superior to simple stenting that further randomization was deemed unethical.[1]

In another randomized study, the positive impact of PDT was confirmed even against those patients in whom adequate biliary drainage could be achieved with stenting alone.[2] It is likely that in the near future PDT will become an integral part of the multidisciplinary treatment of hilar and other forms of CCA in both resectable patients (to improve chances of an R0 resection) as well as in unresectable patients for effective palliation of biliary obstruction.

Brachytherapy

Recently, there has been a resurgence of interest in brachytherapy for the palliation of CCA. I consider brachytherapy in 4 different situations while managing patients with CCA.

If the patient is unresectable but has a relatively localized, small tumor without local extension and no extrahepatic or lymph node metastases, he or she should be considered for liver transplantation based on a recently published Mayo Clinic protocol. This particular protocol incorporates external beam radiation therapy (EBRT), radiation sensitization with 5-FU, low-dose intraluminal brachytherapy (ILBT), and a careful staging laparotomy followed by immediate listing for liver transplant and has been reported to yield a 5-year survival of 82% in carefully selected patients.[3]

The second situation in which to consider palliative brachytherapy is for a patient with completely unresectable CCA as an adjunctive treatment to endoscopic stenting. In these patients, compared to EBRT, brachytherapy is more attractive because it delivers the

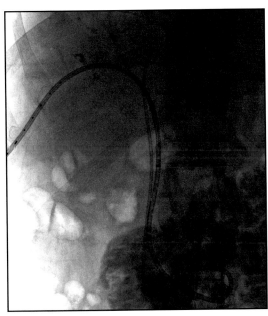

Figure 29-1. Brachytherapy performed through a percutaneous biliary drain. Note the presence of ^{192}Ir seeds within a plastic ribbon passed through the right-sided PBD into position next to the tumor in a patient with CCA. An endoscopic stent is draining the left biliary system.

radiation directly to the target area. Brachytherapy, thus, may be an ideal way to deliver a boost and may allow dose escalation. The reported median survival for patients treated with brachytherapy (with or without EBRT), brachytherapy alone, and no radiation therapy is 11 months, 7 months, and 4 months, respectively.

The third situation where ILBT may be considered is to promote the reduction of risk of recurrent stent occlusion of self-expanding metal stents (SEMS) placed for the palliation of obstructive jaundice caused by CCA.

Lastly, in patients with unresectable intrahepatic CCA, an emerging treatment option is brachytherapy with yttrium-90 radio-embolization, which has been shown to be safe and effective, achieving a partial response in 27% of patients and stabilizing disease in 68% with limited side effects.

In most cases, ILBT is performed in combination with EBRT, which is usually administered in 30 fractions of 150 cGy daily for a total dose of 4500 cGy over 3 weeks along with intravenous 5-FU given on days 1 through 3 as a radiation-sensitizing agent. Intraluminal brachytherapy is delivered by using iridium-192 (^{192}Ir) seeds (half-life of 7 days) placed on a ribbon and mounted on a catheter that is deployed across the tumor by an endoscopic or percutaneous approach (Figure 29-1). The seeds are spaced with a distance of 5 mm from the center of one seed to the other. The ^{192}Ir ribbons are trimmed to the required length and are then threaded into a thin plastic catheter with an embedded radiopaque marker in the tip (Best Industries, Springfield, VA). For hilar CCA, the iridium ribbons can often be placed into the right and left biliary systems in a Y fashion, particularly if the stricture extends more than 1 cm into one or both of the main ducts at the bifurcation. The patient is kept in a shielded inpatient room for 24 hours, and then the catheter is manually removed. Dose rates are typically 50 to 100 cGy per hour at 1.0 cm radius with a total dose of around 2000 to 3000 cGy.[4]

Cholangitis is the most specific complication of ILBT and is reported in up to 6% to 30% of cases. Other related complications are misplacement or migration of the radiation catheter.

Duodenopathy and gastropathy are also common but are related more to the administration of EBRT. I always put these patients on prophylactic proton pump inhibitors (PPIs).

Conclusion

Both PDT and brachytherapy have important roles in the treatment of CCA, particularly when curative intent surgical resection is not a primary option and should be considered in all patients with unresectable tumors for better palliation of cholestasis, improved quality of life, possible prolongation of survival, and, in selected cases, as a neoadjuvant modality prior to a more definitive intervention, such as liver transplantation. These treatment modalities are generally safe. Their main limitation is their lack of local availability given that these therapies are currently available only in few tertiary-care centers of excellence across the country.

References

1. Blechacz B, Gores GJ. Cholangiocarcinoma: advances in pathogenesis, diagnosis, and treatment. *Hepatology.* 2008;48(1):308-321.
2. Berr F. Photodynamic therapy for cholangiocarcinoma. *Semin Liver Dis.* 2004;24(2):177-187.
3. Rea DJ, Heimbach JK, Rosen CB, et al. Liver transplantation with neoadjuvant chemoradiation is more effective than resection for hilar cholangiocarcinoma. *Ann Surg.* 2005;242(3):451-458; discussion 458-461.
4. Simmons DT, Baron TH, Petersen BT, et al. A novel endoscopic approach to brachytherapy in the management of hilar cholangiocarcinoma. *Am J Gastroenterol.* 2006;101(8):1792-1796.

SECTION V

HEPATIC

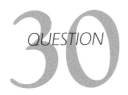

WHAT ARE THE RISK FACTORS FOR THE DEVELOPMENT OF HEPATOCELLULAR CANCER?

Ravinder R. Kurella, MD and William M. Tierney, MD

There are about 8000 new cases of hepatocellular cancer (HCC) diagnosed in the United States each year. Worldwide, HCC accounts for more than 1 million deaths annually and is likely the third most common cause of cancer death.[1] The various risk factors for the development of HCC can be divided into the following categories: chronic viral hepatitis, chronic liver disease other than viral hepatitis, genetic disorders, and dietary and environmental risk factors.

Chronic Viral Hepatitis

Chronic hepatitis B virus (HBV) is the most common cause of HCC worldwide.[2] The risk appears to be related to chronic inflammation as well as the propensity for the viral DNA to insert into hepatocyte DNA and promote mutational carcinogenesis. The absolute risk does appear to be related to the activity of chronic infection, with the active replication state carrying a higher risk than asymptomatic HBsAg-positive carriers. The risk of HCC is much higher in patients who are HBeAg-positive compared to those who are HBsAg-positive but HBeAg-negative. HBV DNA levels correlate with the risk of HCC.[2] Levels of more than 10^5 copies/mL appear to be an independent risk factor for the development of HCC.[2] The relative risk of HCC in the largest prospective study of HBsAg carriers was 223 times that of noncarriers. It is important to realize that in chronic HBV, HCC may occur before cirrhosis develops.

Treatment of hepatitis B does seem to lower the risk of HCC.[3] Successful attainment of a sustained remission in hepatitis B with interferon markedly reduces the rate of HCC. Furthermore, even if a sustained remission is not obtained, the risk of HCC appears to be reduced following therapy. Long-term use of lamivudine in a randomized controlled trial reduced the rate of development of HCC by approximately 2-fold.

While chronic HBV is the most common cause of HCC worldwide, it is chronic hepatitis C virus (HCV) infection that is the most common risk factor for HCC in the United States.[1] Chronic viral hepatitis C-associated HCC generally occurs in the setting of cirrhosis. The prevalence of HCC in noncirrhotic HCV livers appears to be very low.[4] The incidence of HCC tripled in the United States between 1975 and 2005,[1] largely due to the increased prevalence of hepatitis C acquired in the 1960s and 1970s. The incidence of HCC in a HCV-infected patient with cirrhosis is approximately 1% to 7% per year. As with hepatitis B, treatment with interferon does seem to lower the risk of HCC.[5] Co-infection with hepatitis C and hepatitis B appears to result in a higher risk of HCC relative to patients infected with 1 virus.

Chronic Liver Diseases Other Than Viral Hepatitis

There are several chronic liver diseases other than chronic viral hepatitis that may be complicated by HCC. Any form of chronic inflammation that progresses to cirrhosis increases the risk for HCC. Nonalcoholic fatty liver disease (NAFLD) is now the most common chronic liver disease in the United States. It is a clinical and pathological condition, with histology similar to that seen in alcoholic liver disease, but occurs in people who do not drink alcohol. It involves a wide spectrum of histologic findings ranging from simple steatosis to more severe inflammation of the hepatocytes called nonalcoholic steatohepatitis (NASH). Patients with NASH can progress to cirrhosis, and some may develop associated HCC.[6] In addition to NASH, the age of the individual at the time of diagnosis and concurrent alcohol consumption are independent variables for the development of HCC.

Autoimmune hepatitis (AIH) is a chronic progressive inflammatory disease of the liver of unknown etiology. HCC may develop in patients with AIH after progression to cirrhosis but the risk of developing HCC in cirrhotic livers secondary to autoimmune hepatitis is significantly lower when compared to cirrhosis from other causes.

Primary biliary cirrhosis (PBC) is another autoimmune disorder characterized by gradual destruction of small bile ducts by T lymphocytes. HCC occurs with increased frequency in PBC individuals who progress to cirrhosis, although the risk appears to be much lower relative to HCV-related cirrhosis.[7] Older age at the time of diagnosis and male gender is associated with an increased risk of HCC.

Primary sclerosing cholangitis (PSC) is an autoimmune disorder characterized by chronic inflammation and stenosis of the bile ducts and is strongly associated with inflammatory bowel disease. Although cholangiocarcinoma is very common in patients with PSC, there is also an increased incidence of hepatocellular cancer. The prevalence of HCC in patients with cirrhotic PSC is approximately 2%.[8]

Genetic Disorders

Hereditary hemochromatosis is an autosomal recessive disorder of hepatic parenchymal iron overload secondary to excess absorption of dietary iron. It is associated with a markedly increased risk of HCC, as high as 200-fold.[9] The risk of developing HCC could be related to the iron overload itself, because hepatic iron overload in other genetic disorders, such as homozygous Beta thalassemia, is also associated with an increased incidence of HCC. Iron can have a direct effect on cellular proliferation and promote DNA damage, thus causing inactivation of tumor suppressor genes such as p53.

Another recessive disorder, alpha–1-antitripsin (α1-AT) deficiency, is the most common genetic liver disease in infants and children. This disorder is known to cause end-stage liver disease in adults. α1-AT is a serine protease inhibitor that is made primarily in the liver. Its function is to inhibit several proteases. In the absence of α1-AT, these proteases tend to accumulate in the liver and cause hepatocyte injury leading to fibrosis and cirrhosis. Alleles that lead to a reduction in the protein are referred to as deficiency alleles; PiZZ is the most common combination of deficient alleles. Individuals homozygous for this mutation have only 15% of the normal α1-AT levels. PiZZ is the most common genotype leading to cirrhosis and is a risk factor for the development of HCC.

Glycogen storage disorders are rare inborn errors of glycogen metabolism secondary to mutations in the genes encoding various proteins involved in the synthesis of glycogen. There are 12 types of glycogen storage diseases. Types 1 and 3 are associated with an increased risk of hepatocellular adenomas, and there is a risk of subsequent progression to HCC.

Porphyrias are a group of inherited or acquired disorders of enzymes involved in the Heme biosynthetic pathway. Porphyria cutanea tarda (PCT) is the most common subtype of porphyria. The disease is characterized mainly by blistering of sun-exposed portions of the skin. The primary cause of the disorder is deficiency of the enzyme uroporphyrin decarboxylase. PCT is associated with hepatitis C infection and, when occurring together, there is an increased risk of HCC.

Dietary and Environmental Risk Factors

Smoking seems to be an independent risk factor for the development of HCC. People who smoke more than one pack per day have a 5.5-fold increase risk of HCC when compared to nonsmokers or exsmokers.[10] Excessive alcohol intake also has been associated with an increased risk of developing HCC that is approximately twice the risk of smoking. This risk applies particularly to individuals consuming more than 60 g of alcohol a day. Viral hepatitis, alcohol, and smoking appear to have a synergistic effect on the development of HCC. Alcohol also seems to play an additive role in hemochromatosis associated with HCC.

Aflatoxin derived from *Aspergillus flavus*, a mold contaminating stored grains in some parts of the world, increases the risk of HCC in individuals with other risk factors. Mutation of the p53 gene has been demonstrated in patients with HCC who have been chronically exposed to aflatoxin. The risk of developing HCC in patients with HBV who are chronically exposed to aflatoxin is also increased.

Another environmental risk factor associated with HCC is betel quid chewing, often used to produce a stimulant effect in parts of Asia and East Africa. This may be due to aflatoxin contamination as well as the presence of several other potential carcinogens in betel quid. The risk is proportional to the amount and duration of betel quid consumption.

Conclusion

There are numerous environmental and genetic factors that predispose individuals to HCC, and the geographic variation in these risk factors across the world helps to explain the regional disparity of HCC incidence rates. In the United States, chronic liver diseases, including chronic infection with HBV and HCV, are major causes of HCC. Our practice is to focus on the treatment of these disorders with simultaneous modification of patients' lifestyle habits as important means of preventing HCC. It is important to recognize the genetic conditions associated with an increased risk of HCC as specific treatments for some of these disorders may reduce the risk of HCC.

References

1. Altekruse SF, McGlynn KA, Reichman ME. Hepatocellular carcinoma incidence, mortality, and survival trends in the United States From 1975 to 2005. *J Clin Oncol.* 2009;27(9):1485-1491.
2. Chen CJ, Yang HI, Su J, et al. Risk of hepatocellular carcinoma across a biological gradient of serum hepatitis B virus DNA level. *JAMA.* 2006;295(1):65-73.
3. Liaw Y-F, Sung JJ, Chow WC, et al. Lamivudine for patients with chronic hepatitis B and advanced liver disease. *N Engl J Med.* 2004;351(15):1521-1531.
4. Madhoun MF, Fazili J, Bright BC, et al. Hepatitis C prevalence in patients with hepatocellular carcinoma without cirrhosis. *Am J Med Sci.* 2010;339(2):169-173.
5. Lok AS, Seeff LB, Morgan TR, et al. Incidence of hepatocellular carcinoma and associated risk factors in hepatitis C-related advanced liver disease. *Gastroenterology.* 2009;136(1):138-148.
6. Page JM, Harrison SA. Nash and HCC. *Clin Liver Dis.* 2009;13(4):631-647.
7. Farinati F, Floreani A, De Maria N, Fagiuoli S, Naccarato R, Chiaramonte M. Hepatocellular carcinoma in primary biliary cirrhosis. *J Hepatol.* 1994,21(3):315-316.
8. Harnois DM, Gores GJ, Ludwig J, Steers JL, LaRusso NF, Wiesner RH. Are patients with cirrhotic stage primary sclerosing cholangitis at risk for the development of hepatocellular cancer? *J Hepatol.* 1997;27(3):512-516.
9. Kowdley KV. Iron, hemochromatosis, and hepatocellular carcinoma. *Gastroenterology.* 2004;127(5 Suppl 1):S79-S86.
10. Yu MC, Mack T, Hanisch R, Peters RL, Henderson BE, Pike MC. Hepatitis, alcohol consumption, cigarette smoking, and hepatocellular carcinoma in Los Angeles. *Cancer Res.* 1983;43(12 Pt 1):6077-6079.

A 55-YEAR-OLD MAN IS NEWLY DIAGNOSED WITH CIRRHOSIS FROM HEPATITIS C. WHAT IS THE BEST IMAGING MODALITY AND TREATMENT STRATEGY TO SCREEN HIM FOR HEPATOCELLULAR CARCINOMA?

William R. Hutson, MD

Hepatocellular carcinoma (HCC) is one of the most common solid malignancies in the world with an increasing incidence worldwide. During the past decade, HCC has had an exceptional increase in incidence and death rate among solid tumors in the United States. It is postulated that the incidence of HCC will continue to increase for the foreseeable future, primarily due to hepatitis C infection. Most patients with HCC are diagnosed at an advanced stage, which results in a dismal overall 1-year survival rate of only 25% in the United States. Therefore, early detection and treatment of this disease are critical to improve overall clinical outcomes.

Screening is defined as the one-time application of a test that allows detection of asymptomatic disease at a stage when curative intervention may be possible, allowing the goal of reducing morbidity and mortality. We know that screening is effective and has been shown to improve survival in patients with colon, cervical, and breast cancers. The data for screening for HCC are not as convincing, despite the fact that surveillance is widely applied. There is one randomized, controlled trial of surveillance versus no surveillance for HCC that has shown a survival benefit to a strategy of 6-month surveillance with alpha-fetoprotein (AFP) and abdominal ultrasound.[1] This study recruited

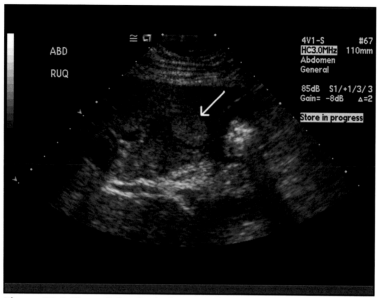

Figure 31-1. Transabdominal ultrasound image of a hyperechogenic mass lesion in the liver in a patient with hepatitis C infection representing hepatocellular carcinoma. The serum AFP was elevated to 368 ng/mL.

18,186 patients in China with current or prior hepatitis B infection. The subjects in the surveillance arm had a reduced mortality related to HCC of 37%. Compliance in the study was poor, so this is probably the minimum benefit to be derived.

There have been decision analysis models that have shown that screening for HCC is a cost-effective strategy. An incidence rate of at least 1.5% per annum should be the starting point for initiating surveillance. The annual incidence rate for patients with hepatitis C virus (HCV)-related HCC is 3.7% to 7.1%. Other high-risk groups for development of HCC include the following: hepatitis B carriers and non-hepatitis B groups with cirrhosis, such as patients with nonalcoholic steatohepatitis (NASH) who have developed cirrhosis, alcoholics, patients with primary biliary cirrhosis, and hereditary hemochromatosis. All of the aforementioned groups are recommended to have screening or surveillance for HCC.

The current recommendations of both the American Association for the Study of Liver Disease (AASLD) and the European Association for the Study of the Liver (EASL) for screening for HCC in the appropriate groups include a serum AFP level and abdominal ultrasound (US). The most commonly used and least expensive screening test for HCC is the serum AFP. Serum AFP levels above 20 ng/mL generally raise concern in high-risk patients. However, sensitivity at this level is relatively poor (41% to 60%), although the specificity of this test is better (80% to 94%). The second most frequently used test for surveillance is transabdominal US. Its performance as a screening test for HCC has been, for the most part, extrapolated from studies that used US as a diagnostic test so its performance as a screening test has not been definitively established. The sensitivity of US for detecting HCC has been shown to be 58% to 78% and the specificity between 93% and 98% (Figure 31-1).

Despite the fact that serum AFP and abdominal US are the official recommendations of the major liver societies, a straw poll taken at the annual AASLD meeting 2 years ago revealed that most hepatologists are selecting magnetic resonance imaging (MRI) or triple-phase computed tomography (CT) scan for screening their patients for HCC. This is a somewhat concerning fact, because there are no objective data to warrant this behavior, and both tests are significantly more expensive than US. CT scans also entail radiation exposure, and in patients who require frequent screening, this can become an issue.

Once an abnormality is detected on a screening test, then a confirmatory test needs to be performed to determine the presence of an HCC. For the diagnosis of HCC, a triple-phase spiral CT or dynamic MRI will typically be chosen. MRI has a sensitivity and specificity of 75% and 76%, respectively, and triple-phase CT scan has a sensitivity and specificity of 61% and 66%, respectively, for the diagnosis of HCC. Other studies have confirmed that MRI is slightly superior to CT scanning for the diagnosis of HCC.[2] In both studies, arterial enhancement of a tumor and delayed washout of contrast is necessary to confirm the likelihood of HCC. Arterial enhancement with delayed washout of a mass in a cirrhotic liver has a sensitivity of about 80%, but a specificity of 95% to 100%. If a lesion does not meet the necessary criteria and there is not an elevated AFP, then a liver biopsy should be performed.[3] However, in practice, it is uncommon to require a biopsy of a lesion, because imaging is usually definitive.

The current guidelines of the AASLD for management of an abnormal screening test for HCC are dictated by the size of the lesion. If a tumor is less than 1 cm in size, then US should be repeated at 3- to 4-month intervals until the lesion is shown to be stable over 18 to 24 months or is shown to be enlarging and then proceed to dynamic imaging studies. If a tumor is between 1 and 2 cm in size, then 2 dynamic imaging studies should be performed. This is because tumors less than 2 cm in size are difficult to characterize and the performance of MRI or CT for small lesions is significantly worse when compared with larger lesions. If a tumor is larger than 2 cm in size, then 1 dynamic imaging study should be used. If there is a typical vascular pattern, then the lesion should be treated as an HCC. If there is an atypical vascular pattern on any of the dynamic imaging studies, then a biopsy of the lesion should be performed.

References

1. Zhang BH, Yang BH, Tang ZY. Randomized controlled trial of screening for hepatocellular carcinoma. *J Cancer Res Clin Oncol.* 2004;130(7):417-422.
2. Rode A, Bancel B, Douek P, et al. Small nodule detection in cirrhotic livers: evaluation with US, spiral CT and MRI and correlation with pathologic examination of explanted liver. *J Comput Assist Tomogr.* 2001;25(3):327-336.
3. Bruix J, Sherman M; Practice Guidelines Committee, American Association for the Study of Liver Diseases. Management of hepatocellular carcinoma. *Hepatology.* 2005;42(5):1208-1236.

WHICH PATIENTS WITH HEPATOCELLULAR CANCER ARE CANDIDATES FOR LIVER TRANSPLANTATION OR SURGICAL RESECTION?

Colin T. Swales, MD and Fredric D. Gordon, MD

Surgical resection or transplant offers the best chance of cure for hepatocellular carcinoma (HCC). One's first thought when approaching a patient with this cancer should be to evaluate whether he or she is a candidate for either of these therapies. Although liver resection is the simplest option, HCC most often occurs in a cirrhotic liver, as cirrhosis is the most prevalent risk factor for HCC. Thus, low hepatic reserve and portal hypertension often make partial hepatic resection unsafe. So, for most patients with HCC, the best option for cure is usually orthotopic liver transplantation (OLT).[1]

Patients with a sporadic HCC (occurring in an otherwise healthy liver), early stage chronic liver disease, or compensated cirrhosis without evidence of portal hypertension may be considered for surgical resection of their lesion. These cases represent the minority of patients with HCC. The anatomic relation of the tumor to major vascular or biliary structures may also preclude their safe resection. For example, a lesion in the middle of the right lobe may require a formal right hepatectomy; a resection this large in a functionally impaired liver would be dangerous as there may be inadequate hepatic reserve to sustain the patient following surgery. On the other hand, a lesion in the left lateral segment in a compensated cirrhotic liver may be appropriate for resection. Impaired liver synthetic function is the usual obstacle to partial hepatic resection, and this should be estimated in advance of any surgical intervention to avoid leaving the patient with too little functioning hepatic tissue following surgery. Liver synthetic function is best measured by the serum albumin, bilirubin, and International Normalized Ratio (INR). An elevated serum bilirubin in the setting of a low serum albumin and an elevated INR suggests poor hepatic synthetic function.

Figure 32-1. Visual representation of the Milan criteria for candidacy for liver transplantation in patients with HCC.

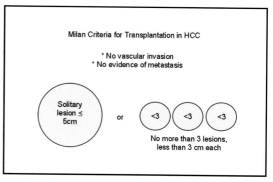

Additional tools to assess the degree of hepatic impairment include the Model for End-Stage Liver Disease (MELD) score, the Child-Turcotte-Pugh (CTP) score, and the presence of portal hypertensive complications including, but not limited to, a history of variceal bleeding and/or the presence of abdominal ascites with a history of spontaneous bacterial peritonitis (SBP). The stress of surgery coupled with the insult to hepatic function may cause hepatic decompensation or worsen any present decompensation, such as ascites or hepatic encephalopathy. Liver decompensation may result in death or could place the patient on a relentless path of a languishing and prolonged debility. A mathematical model, using the MELD score, now exists to predict the risk of death following major surgery in patients with cirrhosis. This risk calculator is derived from prospective data and is available online through the Mayo Clinic Web site (http://www.mayoclinic.org/meld/mayomodel7.html).

Another consideration regarding the best option to treat HCC is the concept of the "field-defect." Because HCC most commonly occurs in a diseased, cirrhotic liver, resecting the known tumor alone still leaves the patient at risk for a new lesion in any remaining hepatic parenchyma. Thus, tumor recurrence may be higher following resection compared with transplantation. Resected patients have 20% to 70% chance of recurrent tumor, compared with 0% to 43% in transplanted patients.[2] These recurrence rates reflect pooled data from cohorts dating back to the 1990s. Recurrence rates following transplant today are far lower, mostly because of better preoperative detection of tumor burden and better selection of candidates for transplantation.

The landmark paper by Mazzaferro and colleagues in 1996 showed that OLT was not only safe, but curative in 90% of cases if patients are carefully chosen.[3] The criteria used in this paper are still used today throughout the world when selecting patients with HCC for liver transplantation. They are known as the Milan criteria and include tumor confined to the liver, without evidence of vascular invasion, a solitary lesion no larger than 5 cm in maximal diameter, or no more than 3 lesions, all of which must be less than 3 cm in maximal diameter (Figure 32-1).

Although not part of the Milan criteria, it is the practice of our center to exclude patients who have a serum alpha-fetoprotein of more than 1000 ng/mL, due to the high likelihood of micro- or macrovascular invasion and subsequent metastatic risk. Other groups have noted the significance of this cutoff as well.

The United Network for Organ Sharing (UNOS) has endorsed OLT as a standard of care for treating HCC within the Milan criteria. Because donor livers are allocated based on the patient's MELD score, patients listed for OLT with HCC are offered "exception points" for having HCC. These points adjust their MELD commensurate with the increased hazard of death caused by having HCC.

There has been a recent movement to expand the bounds of transplantation for HCC, and several centers have published prospective series showing good outcomes in patients who are "beyond Milan criteria" or downstaged into Milan criteria using non-surgical therapies for HCC. The most commonly cited expanded criteria are the UCSF Criteria: a solitary lesion 6.5 cm or less, or 3 or fewer lesions 4.5 cm in maximal diameter or less, total tumor burden 8 cm or less, without evidence of extrahepatic spread or gross vascular invasion. Recently, petitions to UNOS to extend OLT to patients who meet the UCSF criteria have been rejected, as this would further increase organ offers to patients with HCC and disadvantage people without cancer but with a real hazard of death due to cirrhosis who are also in need of liver transplantation.

Last, data have become available showing that preoperative treatment (neoadjuvant treatment) of the HCC improves the outcome of patients with HCC following OLT.[4] Therefore, it has become the policy of our group to treat tumors with either transarterial chemoembolization or radiofrequency ablation, if possible, prior to performing liver transplant. These therapies must be offered in the context of care at a transplant center so that policies set forth by UNOS are followed. Treatment not coordinated with a transplant program may inadvertently disadvantage a patient with HCC or preclude transplantation, thus jeopardizing what is likely the best chance for cure.

References

1. Bruix J, Sherman M. Management of hepatocellular carcinoma. *Hepatology.* 2005;42(5):1208-1236.
2. Llovet JM, Fuster J, Bruix J. Intention-to-treat analysis of surgical treatment for early hepatocellular carcinoma: resection versus transplantation. *Hepatology.* 1999;30(6):1434-1440.
3. Mazzaferro V, Regalia E, Doci R, et al. Liver transplantation for the treatment of small hepatocellular carcinomas in patients with cirrhosis. *N Engl J Med.* 1996;334(11):693-699.
4. Lao OB, Weissman J, Perkins JD. Pre-transplant therapy for hepatocellular carcinoma is associated with a lower recurrence after liver transplantation. *Clin Transplant.* 2009;23(6):874-881.

IN NONSURGICAL PATIENTS WITH HEPATOCELLULAR CANCER, WHAT TREATMENT OPTIONS EXIST, AND HOW EFFECTIVE ARE THEY?

Allene Salcedo Burdette, MD

Hepatocellular carcinoma (HCC) is the fifth most common cancer in men and the eighth most common in women worldwide. Almost 600,000 new cases of HCC are diagnosed annually worldwide. Without therapy, the median length of survival is 6 months, and 5-year survival is a dismal 5%. Transplantation or resection results in the longest survival, but fewer than 20% of patients with HCC are surgical candidates.[1,2]

Several options for liver-directed therapy are available to nonsurgical HCC patients. Because of variation between patients, one treatment is not ideal for all. The method of treatment depends on size, number, and location of the tumor(s); extent of underlying liver disease; and patient performance status. Ideally, before beginning any therapy, a treatment plan for the patient must be delineated. This is most effectively done in a multidisciplinary treatment planning conference.[3]

Historically, the outcome of systemic treatment for HCC has been bleak. Because of rapid innovation and encouraging results with liver-directed therapies, systemic therapies have been mostly relegated to those patients with no other options. With the advent of targeted molecular therapies such as Sorafenib, there has been renewed interest in studying systemic therapies for HCC. Sorafenib, a multikinase inhibitor with antiangiogenic and proapoptotic activity, has been shown to improve overall survival compared with those receiving a placebo.

In an attempt to prolong survival, liver-directed therapy for nonoperative patients should be considered. Options include intra-arterial (IA) therapies and ablative therapies performed by interventional radiologists, and radiation therapy performed by radiation oncologists.

Intra-Arterial Therapies

IA therapy is superior to systemic therapy because a therapeutic agent is delivered selectively into arteries directly supplying the HCC. As a result, therapeutic agents are delivered to the tumor in higher concentrations, resulting in improved therapeutic effect, with less collateral damage to other structures, including adjacent liver parenchyma. This applies to IA therapies that involve embolization. Embolization, in the case of HCC, refers to the occlusion of an artery by injection of various embolic agents, often performed immediately following the administration of a therapeutic agent via IA.

There are 5 methods of IA therapy:

1. Hepatic artery infusion (HAI)

2. Transarterial embolization (TAE)

3. Conventional chemoembolization (cTACE)

4. Drug-eluting bead chemoembolization (DEB-TACE)

5. Radioembolization

With HAI, a subcutaneous infusion port is inserted surgically into the hepatic artery, and 5-FU, doxorubicin, mitomycin C, and other agents, used alone or in combination, are infused into the liver. The tumor is exposed to high concentrations of chemotherapy during the first pass through the liver, but the agent does eventually become systemic. This is not a commonly used modality.

TAE involves the use of embolic agents without chemotherapy or radiation. Embolic agents occlude the feeding arteries of the tumor. This method is not routinely performed because recent literature suggests that ischemia stimulates neoangiogenesis,[1] proliferation, and metastases in HCC, while decreasing chemo- and radiosensitivity. Other literature has demonstrated that even with an initial complete response, the overall survival of those treated with TAE is not changed.

cTACE and DEB-TACE expose HCC to higher concentrations of chemotherapy for a prolonged period of time. Systemic side effects are reduced because the chemotherapy is retained in the liver and is only slowly released into the systemic circulation. Occlusion of the tumor arteries also restricts the flow of oxygen and nutrients to the tumor.[1]

cTACE involves the injection of single or multiple agents into the arterial supply of the tumor. A common mixture consists of cisplatin, doxorubicin, and mitomycin C emulsified with lipiodol, an iodine-containing poppy seed oil. Lipiodol localizes to the HCC, carrying the chemotherapeutic agent with it. Embolization with gelfoam or particles is performed following administration of chemotherapy to increase the dwell time within the tumor.

DEB-TACE is a recent innovation in IA therapy; 100 to 700 μm hydrogel beads loaded with doxorubicin are administered in the same manner as cTACE. DEB-TACE is better tolerated than cTACE due to a more gradual release of chemotherapy systemically. This means higher concentrations of doxorubicin in the tumor for longer periods of time. This effect is more pronounced with DEB-TACE when compared to cTACE. Recent studies show a survival advantage in those treated with DEB-TACE compared with cTACE (Figure 33-1).

Another IA technique is radioembolization or "selective internal radiation therapy" (SIRT). Yttrium-90 (Y-90), a pure beta emitter, is attached to glass or resin microbeads and

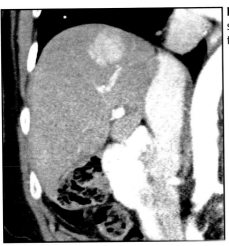

Figure 33-1a. Coronal contrast-enhanced CT demonstrates a hypervascular hepatocellular carcinoma in the dome of the liver.

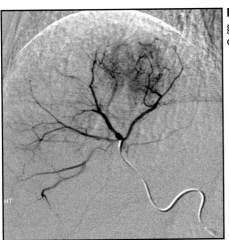

Figure 33-1b. Superselective right hepatic arteriogram demonstrates tumor blush of the hepatocellular carcinoma.

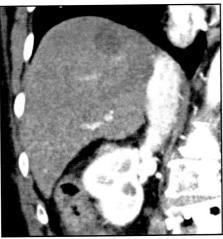

Figure 33-1c. Coronal contrast enhanced CT demonstrates the hepatocellular carcinoma 4 weeks post DEB-TACE. There is no longer arterial enhancement of the lesion.

is injected into the feeding arteries. SIRT is an outpatient procedure and is well-tolerated by patients, with the biggest drawback being fatigue.

With all IA embolization techniques, risks include nontargeted embolization and liver failure. Post-embolization syndrome (pain, elevated white blood cell count, low-grade fever, chills) should be anticipated.[1] Patients typically report fatigue 1 to 2 weeks post-procedure. Complications related to SIRT are potentially more serious than with TACE because of radiation exposure. Non-targeted Y-90 embolization can result in ulceration of an adjacent hollow viscus or radiation-induced liver disease.

Ablative Techniques

Ablative techniques are the second category of liver-directed therapy and can be performed with chemicals or temperature extremes.[4] Ablative techniques produce in situ destruction of tumor tissue, while sparing adjacent non-malignant parenchyma. Guidance for these techniques can be performed with ultrasound, computed tomography (CT), or magnetic resonance imaging (MRI), depending on tumor visibility, with ultrasound being preferred for its real-time capabilities.

Ethanol or acetic acid can be used for chemical ablations (CA). Ethanol works best with smaller lesions, resulting in 90% to 100% necrosis in lesions smaller than 2 cm.[3] Ethanol is less effective at treating adjacent areas of micro-invasion, so the local recurrence rate can be high. The benefits of CA are its simplicity to perform and low cost. Multiple treatments may be necessary when treating larger lesions.[4]

The remaining ablative techniques involve equipment that generates hyperthermia or hypothermia. Radiofrequency ablation (RFA), microwave ablation (MWA), and laser ablation (LA) generate high temperatures within a tumor, resulting in irreversible cellular damage. RFA is the most used ablative technique because of its superior results when compared to CA, especially when treating larger lesions. It is also considered the best therapy for non-operative patients with early stage HCC, with results that rival that of surgical resection (Figure 33-2).[5]

The 2 remaining hyperthermic ablative techniques are microwave (MWA) and laser ablation (LA). With single-probe devices, the areas treated by these modalities are smaller than treatment zones of multi-tined RFA arrays. Development of multi-probe devices will increase the treatment zone size. In treating moderately and poorly differentiated HCCs, MWA has superior overall survival.

Cryoablation has the same indications as RFA. Cryoablation, as compared to RFA, generates a well-characterized region of effect (the "ice ball"), with distinct zones of cellular destruction based upon the distance from the leading edge of the ice ball. Precise sculpting of the ice ball can result in a more defined tumor destruction zone.[4]

One final therapy to consider is radiation therapy (RT). In the past, RT was limited by the development of radiation-induced liver disease (RILD), which depends on the patient's baseline hepatic reserve. New technology allows the focusing of RT doses in a highly conformational manner, resulting in the delivery of higher doses to the tumor while reducing the dose to unaffected parenchyma. Doses up to 90 Gy can be used to safely treat hepatic disease, if the volume of irradiated liver is kept to a minimum.[5] Stereotactic body radiation therapy (SBRT) and 3-dimensional conformal radiotherapy (3D-CRT) are 2 methods that have been used alone or in conjunction with TACE to treat nonsurgical HCC patients.

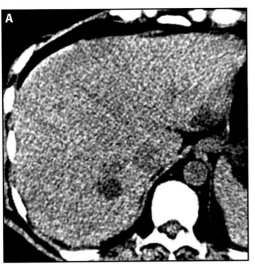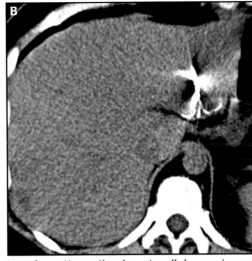

Figure 33-2. (A) Unenhanced axial CT demonstrates a low attenuation hepatocellular carcinoma in the left hepatic lobe. A second lesion is noted in the right hepatic lobe, which is to be resected surgically. (B) Unenhanced axial CT demonstrates a multi-tined RFA array deployed percutaneously in the left hepatic hepatocellular carcinoma.

Conclusion

Overall, patients with intact liver function, good performance status, and early tumor stage do best regardless of the chosen treatment modality. Survival rate decreases and morbidity increases as these parameters decline.[3] Many treatment options exist for the nonoperative HCC population, with different outcomes depending on patient and tumor characteristics. To customize patient care, one has to take these variables into account, and the best option should be determined after extensive discussion in a multidisciplinary treatment conference.

References

1. Brown D, Geschwind J, Soulen M, Millward SF, Sacks D. Society of Interventional Radiology position statement on chemoembolization of hepatic malignancies. *J Vasc Interv Radiol.* 2009;20(7 Suppl):S317-S323.
2. Varela M, Sala M, Llovet JM, Bruix J. Treatment of hepatocellular carcinoma: is there an optimal strategy? *Cancer Treat Rev.* 2003;29(2):99-104.
3. Bruix J, Sherman M; Practice Guidelines Committee, American Association for the Study of Liver Diseases. Management of hepatocellular carcinoma. *Hepatology.* 2005;42(5):1208-1236.
4. Barnett CC, Curley SA. Ablation techniques: ethanol injection, cryoablation, and radiofrequency ablation. *Operative Techniques in General Surgery.* 2002;4(1):65-75.
5. Hawkins MA, Dawson LA. Radiation therapy for hepatocellular carcinoma, from palliation to cure. *Cancer.* 2006;106(8):1653-1663.

A 67-Year-Old Woman With Cirrhosis Develops Hepatocellular Cancer. Shortly After Diagnosis, She Becomes Jaundiced. How Do You Determine if the Jaundice Is Due to Cirrhosis, Biliary Obstruction, or Both?

Darryn Potosky, MD and Eric Goldberg, MD

Jaundice is yellow discoloration of the skin as a result of increased serum bilirubin levels. Cholestasis is a pathologic state in which the flow of bile from the liver to the intestines is impaired and can result from intrahepatic dysfunction or extrahepatic obstruction. In patients with cirrhosis, intrahepatic cholestasis can result from a progressive decline in hepatic function or a super-imposed insult to the liver, such as acute viral hepatitis, portal or hepatic venous occlusion, sepsis, drug injury, or alcoholic hepatitis. While most patients with cirrhosis will develop jaundice during the course of their illness, they can also develop extrahepatic biliary obstruction as a result of gallstones, benign strictures, or malignancy. As the differential diagnosis of jaundice in the patient with cirrhosis is broad, it may be challenging to determine the exact etiology.

The development of hepatocellular carcinoma can cause decompensation of a previously stable cirrhotic liver, leading to worsening hyperbilirubinemia. It is less common to have a hepatoma cause biliary obstruction unless it is large or directly invading the bile duct (Figure 34-1). A case series by Wang and colleagues[1] evaluated 491 patients

Figure 34-1. Multifocal hepatocellular carcinoma with focal dilation of the ductal system in the left lobe.

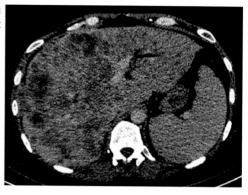

with biopsy-proven hepatocellular carcinoma. Out of these patients, only 9 (1.8%) had dilated bile ducts with evidence of tumor thrombi within the ducts. Eight patients had tumor infiltrating into and obstructing adjacent major bile ducts. While this complication was uncommon, it is important to remember that cirrhotic patients can develop biliary obstruction from any cause similar to the noncirrhotic population. Therefore, one must be vigilant to fully evaluate all cirrhotic patients with new hyperbilirubinemia for potential obstruction, rather than simply attribute it to worsening of the underlying disease.

Evaluation of the Patient

The initial assessment of the cirrhotic patient with cholestasis is based on a thorough history, physical examination, and serum liver chemistries. Acute biliary obstruction often presents with abdominal pain, frequently in the right upper quadrant, whereas this would be an uncommon symptom of intrahepatic cholestasis. The presence of fever should raise the clinical suspicion for ascending cholangitis, most commonly due to stone disease. In general, rapid development of jaundice often indicates an obstructive process where a more insidious onset is often seen with intrahepatic cholestasis. The physical exam may reveal a palpable liver mass or gallbladder, which may be helpful in differentiating the cause of jaundice. More often, examination will only show stigmata of chronic liver disease that will not help guide further evaluation.

While routine liver chemistries will often fail to definitively distinguish intrahepatic from extrahepatic cholestasis, they may offer subtle clues that can be useful for the clinician. Initial laboratory evaluation should include fractionation of the bilirubin. A predominance of unconjugated bilirubin should alert the clinician to the presence of hemolysis, whereas patients with extrahepatic obstruction will have a majority of the conjugated fraction. Unfortunately, this is not useful in distinguishing the type of cholestasis, as conjugated hyperbilirubinemia is also seen with intrahepatic cholestasis. A marked elevation in the serum alkaline phosphatase level from the patient's baseline may suggest extrahepatic obstruction. The degree and ratio of serum aminotransferase elevation does not assist in this differential with the exception of levels greater than 1000 U/L, which often suggests a toxic, infectious, or ischemic injury to the liver. While an increase in the prothrombin time can be seen with a progressive decline in liver function, it may also result from impaired absorption of fat-soluble vitamins secondary to inadequate amounts of bile in the duodenum. Vitamin K administration will not normalize the prothrombin times of patients with hepatic dysfunction and intrahepatic cholestasis but will improve the prothrombin time in patients with extrahepatic obstruction.

Imaging Studies

Imaging of the liver and biliary system is often necessary to distinguish intrahepatic cholestasis from extrahepatic obstruction. When intra- or extrahepatic ductal dilation is present, it strongly suggests the presence of obstruction. Anecdotally, ductal dilation may not be a prominent feature in the cirrhotic liver because fibrosis can impede dilation. Therefore, the absence of ductal dilation does not always exclude an obstruction. This also becomes an issue in the post-transplant setting where one may not see a dilated ductal system even in the presence of a high-grade anastomotic stricture.

A right upper quadrant ultrasound with Doppler is often the first imaging test employed. In addition to detecting ductal dilation, stones, and the presence of tumor, it can also exclude hepatic or portal venous obstruction or thrombosis. While ultrasound can demonstrate cholelithiasis easily, it is much less sensitive for common bile duct stones (choledocholithiasis) due to overlying bowel gas in the duodenum.

Contrast-enhanced CT scans are more sensitive for evaluation of the biliary system than ultrasound and will also provide a comprehensive view of the liver and surrounding tissues. CT may still not be sensitive for distal bile duct stones and has a lower sensitivity for gallbladder stones than ultrasound. Additionally, this requires contrast, which can be nephrotoxic and involves the use of ionizing radiation.

Magnetic resonance cholangiopancreatography (MRCP) provides detailed imaging of the biliary tree and pancreatic duct. In patients with dilated ducts, MRCP is diagnostic in more than 90% of patients, almost always reveals the level of obstruction, and has a 90% to 100% sensitivity and specificity for choledocholithiasis and biliary strictures.[2] MRCP is not only helpful for determining whether there is obstruction, but it can also guide which bile ducts drain in order to provide palliation.[3] For example, in a patient with multifocal hepatocellular carcinoma where one lobe of the liver has extensive disease and the other has a focal obstruction, the MRCP will guide which lobe will be most beneficial to drain. Furthermore, contrast injection into the lobe of the liver that will not benefit from drainage can be avoided, reducing the development of infectious complications after endoscopic retrograde cholangiopancreatography (ERCP). Limitations of MRCP include expense, patient factors such as the inability to breath hold or remain still, the presence of metallic objects (pacemaker, automated implantable cardioverter-defibrillator [AICD]), and the technology and expertise of the center performing the study.

Interventions

In cases where the findings on MRCP are equivocal, ERCP is the gold standard for determining the presence of an obstruction in the biliary system. Additionally, when there is a high expectation of biliary obstruction at the outset, we would proceed directly to ERCP, as a negative imaging study would not preclude the subsequent performance of ERCP. While the risks of ERCP are inherently higher than any of the imaging tests

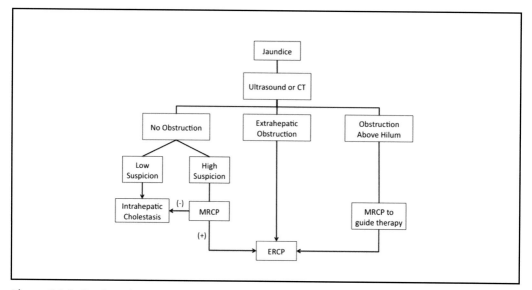

Figure 34-2. Our imaging approach to distinguishing intrahepatic cholestasis from extrahepatic obstruction.

mentioned, its ability to provide therapy is essential, especially when urgent decompression of the bile duct is needed. In cases where the ducts may not be dilated (cirrhosis and post-transplant), ERCP may be the only test to demonstrate the site of obstruction. If ERCP is unsuccessful, consideration can be given to the placement of a percutaneous biliary drain.

Our approach to the patient with new-onset jaundice in the setting of hepatocellular carcinoma who may have a biliary obstruction is outlined in Figure 34-2. It is important to remember that jaundice in these patients is often multifactorial. When biliary obstruction is present with cirrhosis, relieving the obstruction will improve the hyperbilirubinemia, but often only back to the patient's previous baseline values.

References

1. Wang JH, Chen TM, Tung HD, Lee CM, Changchien CS, Lu SN. Color Doppler sonography of bile duct tumor thrombi in hepatocellular carcinoma. *J Ultrasound Med.* 2002;21(7):767-772.
2. Saini S. Imaging of the hepatobiliary tract. *N Engl J Med.* 1997;336(26):1889.
3. Freeman ML, Overby C. Selective MRCP and CT-targeted drainage of malignant hilar biliary obstruction with self-expanding metallic stents. *Gastrointestinal Endosc.* 2003;58(1):41-49.

A 55-Year-Old Man With Cirrhosis Is Found to Have a 1.5-cm Liver Lesion and an Elevated Alpha-Fetoprotein. Is a Biopsy or Other Testing Required to Confirm a Diagnosis of Hepatocellular Carcinoma? What Other Evaluation Is Warranted?

Fredric D. Gordon, MD

Hepatocellular carcinoma is the sixth most common cancer and the third leading cause of cancer deaths worldwide. It is estimated that, in the United States, the number of cases of hepatocellular carcinoma will increase by 81% over the current baseline of 13,000 cases per year by the year 2020. Most of this increase is attributable to the rising prevalence of hepatitis C cirrhosis. The risk factors for the development of hepatocellular carcinoma are listed in Table 35-1.[1]

The patient described in this question provides some interesting diagnostic considerations. He is certainly in a high-risk group based on the presence of cirrhosis as well as his age and gender. Although we are not given the cause of his cirrhosis, we may statistically presume that it is due to excessive alcohol use and/or hepatitis C, both of which are risk factors for hepatocellular carcinoma. My approach to a liver mass in a cirrhotic patient is to assume that the lesion is hepatocellular carcinoma until proven otherwise. There are data to suggest that more than 80% of masses larger than 2 cm in size in a cirrhotic

> ## Table 35-1
> # Risk Factors for the Development of Hepatocellular Carcinoma
>
> - Cirrhosis of any cause
> - Noncirrhotic chronic hepatitis B
> - Excessive alcohol consumption
> - Hereditary hemochromatosis
> - Older age
> - Male gender
> - Family history of hepatocellular carcinoma

liver are hepatocellular carcinoma. Furthermore, there are additional data to suggest that 75% of masses under 2 cm in size in a cirrhotic liver are also hepatocellular carcinomas. Other diagnostic considerations in the cirrhotic liver include dysplastic nodule, regenerative nodule, cholangiocarcinoma, hepatic lymphoma, hemangioma, hepatic adenoma, metastasis, and focal nodular hyperplasia.[2]

The patient in question has an elevated alpha-fetoprotein (AFP). First, it is important to note that 20% of all patients with hepatocellular carcinoma and 30% of patients with small hepatocellular carcinomas (less than 2 cm) will have a persistently normal AFP. Conversely, an AFP higher than 200 to 400 ng/mL is virtually diagnostic of hepatocellular carcinoma in the absence of acute hepatitis; however, this level of AFP is only found in 18% to 20% of patients with hepatocellular carcinoma. An AFP higher than 1000 ng/mL correlates with a poor prognosis and increased likelihood of vascular invasion (61%). Studies evaluating the role of AFP as a screening test in an at-risk population show that a cutoff value of 20 ng/mL provides the best balance between sensitivity and specificity, at 62% and 89%, respectively. In a population whose risk for hepatocellular carcinoma is 50% (as might be expected in our patient), an AFP higher than 20 ng/mL confers a positive predictive value of 85%. An AFP higher than 100 ng/mL increases the positive predictive value to more than 96%.

In our patient with an "elevated serum AFP," a level higher than 400 ng/mL would therefore be diagnostic of hepatocellular carcinoma, and a biopsy would be unnecessary. A level between 20 and 400 ng/mL would be strongly suggestive of hepatocellular carcinoma but not yet diagnostic.

The American Association for the Study of Liver Diseases (AASLD) has developed an algorithm[3] that is useful for the evaluation of an undiagnosed liver mass in the setting of cirrhosis. If the lesion is less than 1 cm in size, the likelihood of hepatocellular carcinoma is extremely small, and further radiologic surveillance with ultrasound every 3 to 4 months is appropriate. If the lesion is stable over 18 to 24 months, then routine surveillance every 6 to 12 months can continue.

Alternatively, if the lesion grows or is initially found to be 1 to 2 cm in size, then the risk of hepatocellular carcinoma is higher. In that case, 2 dynamic, cross-sectional studies (ie, triphasic computed tomography [CT] scan and contrast-enhanced MRI) should be performed. If both studies agree that the lesion is consistent with hepatocellular carcinoma, then the diagnosis is confirmed, and a biopsy is not necessary. If either or both studies demonstrate an atypical radiographic pattern for hepatocellular carcinoma, then biopsy of the lesion should be performed.

I believe this recommendation to biopsy should be interpreted with caution for several reasons:

- There is a 2% to 3% risk of seeding the biopsy tract with hepatocellular carcinoma.
- There may be relative or absolute contraindications to biopsy, such as severe coagulopathy or ascites.
- There is a clinically significant false-negative rate.

For patients in whom the decision to defer biopsy is made, serial monitoring of the alpha-fetoprotein and contrast-enhanced cross-sectional imaging every 3 months is a suitable alternative. I also have a slightly lower threshold to biopsy the lesion if the AFP is normal because the possibility of primary hepatic lymphoma would demand a radically different treatment approach. The AASLD also recommends that for lesions greater than 2 cm in size, a single dynamic imaging study demonstrating typical features of hepatocellular carcinoma or an alpha-fetoprotein level higher than 200 ng/mL is diagnostic of hepatocellular carcinoma. If neither of these criteria is met, then biopsy (or the alternative monitoring offered above) is appropriate.

According to the AASLD guidelines, the 55-year-old patient in question should undergo 2 dynamic imaging studies. Standard ultrasound is usually inadequate to definitively diagnose hepatocellular carcinoma. The addition of Doppler ultrasound can increase the specificity when a portal vein thrombosis is found in association with a parenchymal mass. Contrast-enhanced, phasic (at least late arterial phase and portal venous phase) cross-sectional imaging with CT or MRI can increase the sensitivity to approximately 90% and specificity to approximately 95%. Hepatocellular carcinomas are typically hypervascular and, therefore, enhance in the arterial phase (hyperdense on CT and hyperintense on T2-weighted MRI images). This hypervascularity also results in more rapid washout of contrast (hypodense and hypointense) in the portal venous phase compared to the surrounding liver parenchyma. In addition, the findings of late (pseudo) capsule enhancement and interval growth on serial imaging also strongly suggest hepatocellular carcinoma.

In 2009, a national conference was convened under the auspices of the Organ Procurement and Transplantation Network (OPTN)/United Network for Organ Sharing (UNOS) and other transplantation societies. The conference addressed the radiologic criteria for the diagnosis of hepatocellular carcinoma and developed a classification system for nodules on imaging of cirrhotic livers (Table 35-2). In addition to clarifying diagnostic radiologic criteria for hepatocellular carcinoma, recommendations for follow-up studies for indeterminate lesions are made.[4]

A few key points to remember:

- It is highly likely that this patient has hepatocellular carcinoma (at least a 75% chance).
- There is no urgency to make this diagnosis today; the lesion has been there for weeks or months. Hepatocellular carcinomas typically grow slowly so making an accurate diagnosis today or in 2 to 4 weeks will have no impact on the treatment options.
- A careful and precise diagnosis is essential to provide the proper care for the patient.

Table 35-2
Organ Procurement and Transplantation Network

Class	Description	Comment
0	Incomplete or technically inadequate study	Repeat study is required for adequate assessment; automatic priority MELD points cannot be assigned on the basis of an OPTN class 0 classified imaging study.
1	No evidence of HCC on good-quality, appropriate surveillance examination	Typically, surveillance would continue according to the routine practice at the respective transplant center.
2	Benign lesion(s) or diffuse parenchymal abnormality with no dominant focal lesion	Typically, the need for any further imaging would be determined on a clinical basis according to the routine practice at the respective transplant center (MRI preferred over CT).
3	Abnormal scan, indeterminate focal lesion(s), not currently meeting radiological criteria for HCC	Typically, follow-up imaging would be performed in 6 to 12 months (MRI preferred over CT).
4	Abnormal scan, intermediate suspicion for HCC (meets some radiological criteria for HCC and could represent HCC)	Consider short-term follow-up in 3 (maximum diameter of lesions 2 cm) to 6 months (maximum diameter of lesions < 2 cm), with MRI preferred over CT or biopsy. Imaging follow-up should be considered if biopsy is negative or not possible.
5	Meets radiological criteria for HCC	Patient may be eligible for automatic priority MELD points on the basis of this imaging study. Please refer to definitions for class 5 criteria.

Reprinted with permission from Pomfret EA, Washburn K, Wald C, et al. Report of a national conference on liver allocation in patients with hepatocellular carcinoma in the United States. *Liver Transplantation*. 2010;16:262-278.

References

1. Shariff MIF, Cox IJ, Gomea AI, Khan SA, Gedroyc W, Taylor-Robinson SD. Hepatocellular carcinoma: current trends in worldwide epidemiology, risk factors, diagnosis, and therapeutics. *Expert Rev Gastroenterol Hepatol.* 2009;3(4):353-367.
2. Assy N, Nasser G, Djibre A, Beniashvili Z, Elias S, Zidan J. Characteristics of common solid liver lesions and recommendations for diagnostic workup. *World J Gastroenterol.* 2009;15(26):3217-3227.
3. Bruix J, Sherman M; Practice Guidelines Committee, American Association for the Study of Liver Diseases. Management of hepatocellular carcinoma. *Hepatology.* 2005;42(5):1208-1236.
4. Pomfret EA, Washburn K, Wald C, et al. Report of a national conference on liver allocation in patients with hepatocellular carcinoma in the United States. *Liver Transplantation.* 2010;16(3):262-278.

SECTION VI

SMALL BOWEL AND COLON

WHICH DISEASES INCREASE THE RISK OF DEVELOPING SMALL BOWEL CARCINOMA?

Caroline R. Tadros, MD

Despite the fact that the small intestine comprises 75% of the gastrointestinal (GI) tract, small intestinal neoplasms only account for 1% to 2% of all GI malignancies. Approximately two-thirds of these neoplasms are malignant. It has been hypothesized that this low rate of malignancy is due to a combination of the following:

- The rapid transit time of luminal contents within the small bowel (decreases mucosal contact with potential carcinogens)
- The low bacterial count
- Rapid epithelial cell turnover (leads to shedding of mutation-carrying cells)
- Local lymphoid tissue, which plays a role in surveillance of malignancy
- The presence of detoxifying enzymes such as mucosal hydrolases (which may work to convert carcinogens into less toxic substances within the lumen).[1]

The increased intraluminal pH may also prevent the formation of nitrosamines, which typically form in acidic environments. These agents have been associated with gastric malignancies. Therefore, diseases or environmental factors that alter these parameters may be associated with an increased risk of malignancy.[1,2]

Epidemiology and Risk Factors

According to the National Cancer Database,[3] there were 1110 deaths and 6230 new cases of small intestinal cancer in the United States in 2009. Most of these cancers occur in patients over the age of 60, and there is a higher incidence in African Americans. The majority of these lesions occur proximally, with approximately 50% to 60% occurring within the duodenum, 18% to 22% in the jejunum, and 10% to 15% in the ileum.[2]

Figure 36-1. Endoscopic image of small-bowel adenocarcinoma in an 81-year-old male. (Reprinted with permission of Douglas G. Adler, MD.)

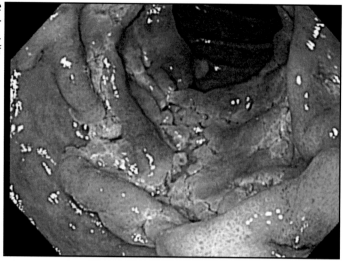

The most commonly occurring small intestinal neoplasms are adenocarcinomas, sarcomas (GI stromal tumors [GISTs]), carcinoids, and lymphomas. Adenocarcinoma is the most common primary small intestinal neoplasm accounting for approximately 35% to 50% of all lesions (Figure 36-1). Carcinoids are the second most common lesion, accounting for between 20% and 40%. Lymphomas and sarcomas each account for approximately 14%.[2]

The histopathology of small intestinal neoplasms is quite varied due to the fact that they can arise from all of the cell lines that comprise the small intestine. They can originate from mucosal glands, smooth muscle, argentaffin cells, nerve sheaths, fibroblasts, neurons, mesenchymal cells, lymphocytes, or vascular structures. The distribution of neoplasms within the bowel varies with their cellular origin. Small intestinal lymphomas and carcinoids are most commonly found within the ileum. More than half of all adenocarcinomas occur in the duodenum; and, of those, approximately 60% are adjacent to the ampulla. This suggests that bile and/or pancreatic juice may have an oncogenic effect on the small intestinal mucosa.[1] Sarcomas tend to be more evenly distributed; however, there is a slight predilection in the jejunum.[2]

Wu and colleagues[1] investigated the role of alcohol, tobacco, and diet in the development of small intestinal adenocarcinoma. Prior case-controlled studies demonstrated that consumption of red meat and heterocyclic amines (typically found in smoked, barbecued, or salted foods) were associated with an increased risk of small intestinal cancer. These investigators performed a large population-based case-control study of multisite cancers in Los Angeles County between 1975 and 1984. Thirty-six patients with histologically proven small intestinal adenocarcinoma were identified and were compared to 998 controls. They found that heavy alcohol consumption (more than 80 g a day) and a high daily intake of sugar were strong risk factors in both men and women. Cigarette smoking and intake of heterocyclic amines were only associated with an increased risk in men. African American ethnicities have also been demonstrated to be a major risk factor for the development of malignancy, but the reasons for this are unclear.

Inflammatory conditions such as Crohn's disease and celiac sprue have been associated with an increased risk of small intestinal cancer. Patients with small intestinal

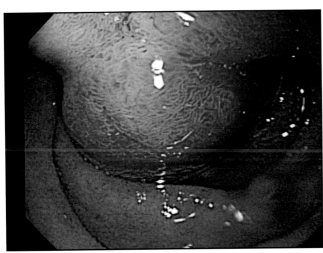

Figure 36-2. Malignant mass in the small bowel in a patient with Peutz-Jeghers syndrome. (Reprinted with permission of Douglas G. Adler, MD.)

Crohn's disease have a 6-fold higher rate of adenocarcinoma than the general population.[4] Longstanding inflammation leads to dysplasia and ultimately carcinoma.[5] Small intestinal cancers associated with Crohn's disease typically occur in the distal jejunum and ileum, whereas sporadic cancers tend to occur in the duodenum.[4] The 2-year survival rate of small bowel adenocarcinoma is between 15% and 23%; however, when it occurs in the setting of Crohn's disease, the 2-year survival rate drops to less than 10%.[4]

Male patients with a longstanding history of Crohn's disease, especially fistulizing or poorly controlled disease, have the highest risk of developing small bowel cancer. Longer disease duration and history of bowel resection have also been identified as independent risk factors; however, the extent to which each of these factors increases the risk remains unclear. Adenocarcinoma, carcinoids, and lymphomas have all been associated with areas of active inflammation in Crohn's disease. It also remains unclear as to what causes the development of lymphoma in these patients.[4]

Celiac sprue has been associated with esophageal, oropharyngeal, and small intestinal carcinomas. Small intestinal lymphoma accounts for 50% to 60% of the malignancies associated with celiac disease, and these usually develop after 20 to 40 years of disease duration. This lymphoma is of T-cell origin, whereas small intestinal lymphoma that occurs in the general population often arises from B-cell lines, although both B- and T-cell lymphoma can be seen in celiac patients. This is an aggressive disease with a 5-year survival rate of approximately 11%.[2]

Patients with polyposis syndromes such as familial adenomatous polyposis (FAP), hereditary nonpolyposis colorectal cancer (HNPCC), and Peutz-Jeghers syndrome have a high risk of developing small intestinal adenocarcinoma (Figure 36-2). These small bowel adenocarcinomas progress through the adenoma-carcinoma sequence. In FAP, small bowel adenocarcinoma is the leading cause of death in patients who have undergone colectomy. These neoplasms typically occur adjacent to the ampulla of Vater and tend to be larger with more advanced histology. They are more likely to undergo malignant transformation than neoplasms located elsewhere in the bowel. Patients with Peutz-Jeghers syndrome develop hamartomatous polyps throughout the small and large intestine; however, these lesions most commonly occur within the jejunum. These polyps result from mutations in the LKB1 gene, which encodes a serine threonine kinase.[2]

In addition to the major risk factors of Crohn's and celiac disease, there are many minor risk factors for the development of small intestinal neoplasms. Cholecystectomy and a history of radiation have been associated with an increase the risk of carcinoma. Patients with HIV/AIDS have an increased risk of lymphoma. Anal cancer, a high-fat diet, squamous cell skin cancer, Wilm's tumor, and Hodgkins lymphoma have all been identified as minor risk factors for the development of small bowel neoplasms.[2]

Surgical resection is the only option to cure malignant small bowel adenocarcinoma. In patients with Crohn's disease, control of inflammation through the use of immunomodulators or biologics decreases the risk of adenocarcinoma. There has been debate as to whether or not the use of immunomodulators increases the risk of lymphoma in this population. Treatment of small bowel inflammation in celiac disease requires strict adherence to a gluten-free diet. CT or capsule endoscopy should be performed in celiac patients with previously well-controlled disease who suddenly develop abdominal pain, weight loss, or diarrhea despite maintaining a gluten-free diet. Patients with familial polyposis syndromes should be enrolled in aggressive endoscopic surveillance programs and possible capsule endoscopy to detect high-risk lesions.

References

1. Wu AH, Yu MC, Mack TM. Smoking, alcohol use, dietary factors and risk of small intestinal adenocarcinoma. *Int J Cancer.* 1997;70(5):512-517.
2. Rustgi AK. Small intestinal neoplasms. In: Feldman M, Friedman LS, Brandt LJ, eds. *Sleisinger and Fordtran's Gastrointestinal and Liver Diseases: Pathophysiology, Diagnosis, Management.* 8th ed. Ontario, Canada: Saunders; 2006:2703-2712.
3. National Cancer Institute. PDQ: NCI's Comprehensive Cancer Database. Bethesda, MD: US National Institutes of Health, 2010. http://www.cancer.gov/cancertopics/types/smallintestine. Accessed March 2010.
4. Bernstein D, Rogers A. Malignancy in Crohn's disease. *Am J Gastorenterol.* 1996;91(3):434-440.
5. Mizushima T, Ohno Y, Nakajima K, et al. Malignancy in Crohn's disease: incidence and clinical characteristics in Japan. *Digestion.* 2010;81(4):265-270.

What Are the Current Guidelines for Screening for Colorectal Cancer?

Harshinie C. Amaratunge, MD and Waqar A. Qureshi, MD

In the United States, colorectal cancer (CRC) is the third most common type of cancer and the second leading cause of cancer death. There is good evidence that screening individuals greater than 50 years of age reduces colorectal cancer mortality. There are several screening tests that can be used for primary screening of average-risk adults. The following screening tests are currently available:

- Endoscopy (colonoscopy and flexible sigmoidoscopy)
- Radiological imaging (computed tomography [CT] colonography and double-contrast barium enema)
- Stool tests (DNA, hemoccult, high-sensitivity hemoccult, and immunochemical tests)

Several medical societies have developed guidelines for screening strategies based on the currently available screening tests. Until mid-2008, all guidelines recommended any one of the screening tests and strategies based on patient preference, cost-effectiveness, and availability. In 2008, updated guidelines were published by 2 major guideline organizations: The Joint "multi-society" guidelines[1] (an aggregation of the American Cancer Society [ACS], the Multi-Society Task Force [MSTF], which consists of the American Gastroenterological Association, American Society of Gastrointestinal Endoscopy, the American College of Gastroenterology, and the American College of Radiology [ACR]) and the guideline from the US Preventive Services Task Force (USPSTF).[2] One of the key differences between these 2 guidelines concerns the recommendation of the newer modalities of CT colonography (CTC) and fecal DNA testing; the USPSTF feels that there is insufficient evidence to endorse these 2 tests.

At this time, the *USPSTF 2008* recommends that primary screening for colon cancer for average-risk adults should begin at age 50 and continue until age 75 years. These recommendations do not apply to those patients with a specific inherited cancer syndrome or inflammatory bowel disease (who require more intensive screening). Screening can be accomplished with annual high-sensitivity fecal occult blood test (FOBT), Sensa or fecal immunochemical test (FIT), sigmoidoscopy every 5 years with high-sensitivity FOBT every 3 years, or colonoscopy every 10 years. USPSTF recommends against routine screening for CRC in adults ages 76 to 85 years and against screening in those older than 85 years. The likelihood of early adenoma detection and endoscopic or surgical intervention yields a significant mortality benefit due to the average (and lengthy) amount of time between adenoma development and cancer diagnosis.

The *Joint Guideline* stresses that patient preferences and availability of resources play an important role in the selection of screening tests. Colon cancer prevention should be the primary goal of CRC screening. Tests that are designed to detect both early cancer and adenomatous polyps should be encouraged. These test include flexible sigmoidoscopy every 5 years, colonoscopy every 10 years, double contrast barium enema (DCBE) every 5 years, or CTC every 5 years. Tests that primarily detect cancer are annual FOBT or FIT. Fecal DNA testing is also recommended; however, the interval at which to repeat the test is uncertain. In addition, most physicians have no experience in ordering (or interpreting) fecal DNA testing.

The *American Cancer Society Guideline for Early Detection of Cancer* specifically states that average-risk adults begin screening using one of the following 5 options: annual FOBT or FIT, flexible sigmoidoscopy every 5 years,[3] flexible sigmoidoscopy plus FOBT/FIT every 5 years, colonoscopy every 10 years, or double-contrast barium enema every 5 years.

ACS and USPSTF found that there was insufficient evidence to recommend one test over another based on the balance of potential benefits, cost-effectiveness, potential harms, and also the variability in access and patient choice.

The American College of Gastroenterology's (ACG) 2008 updated practice guideline stresses that screening tests should be divided into cancer prevention and cancer detection.[4] A cancer prevention test is preferred over a detection test. The college also endorses a preferred strategy for screening compared to a list of possible options that have been recommended from the other societies. For primary screening, the ACG states that a colonoscopy every 10 years is the preferred CRC prevention test for patients aged 50 and older. Importantly, the college endorses the notion that, for Blacks, screening should begin at age 45 years due to increased overall risk. Alternative CRC prevention tests include flexible sigmoidoscopy every 5 to 10 years or CT colonography every 5 years. If a patient declines colonoscopy or another CRC prevention test, then a cancer detection test should be offered. The preferred cancer detection test in this situation is annual FIT to detect occult bleeding. Alternative CRC detection tests include annual Hemoccult Sensa or fecal DNA testing every 3 years. ACG does not make recommendations regarding at what age screening should no longer be considered, but some fit elderly individuals are screened well into their eighties.

The *Joint Guideline* also provides recommendations regarding those individuals at an increased risk compared to average-risk individuals. In patients with a first-degree relative with colorectal cancer or adenomatous polyps before age 60 years or 2 or more first-degree relatives at any age, screening with colonoscopy should begin at age 40 or 10 years before the youngest case in the immediate family. Colonoscopy should thereafter be repeated every 5 years. In a patient with a first-degree relative with colorectal cancer diagnosed at less than age 60 or in second-degree relatives with CRC, screening should begin at age 40 years with either of the screening strategies available for average-risk individuals. However, the ACG recommends average-risk screening for an individual with a single first-degree relative with CRC or advanced adenoma diagnosed at an age older than 60 years.

Above-average risk individuals include those with the following conditions:

- Familial adenomatous polyposis (FAP) and attenuated FAP
- Hereditary nonpolyposis coli (HNPCC)
- Inflammatory bowel disease
- Personal history of colon cancer or adenomatous polyps
- Colon cancer or adenomatous polyps in first-degree relatives.

Individuals with a diagnosis of FAP should start screening at age 10 to 12 years with annual flexible sigmoidoscopy, and early colectomy should be considered. For individuals with a diagnosis of HNPCC, colonoscopy every 1 to 2 years should be performed starting at age 20 to 25 years or 10 years before the youngest case of colorectal cancer in the immediate family. For patients with inflammatory bowel disease, screening should start 8 years after the onset of pancolitis and 12 to 15 years after the onset of left-sided colitis with colonoscopy and biopsies. This should be repeated every 1 to 2 years. As described above, the consensus among the different guideline committees is that colon cancer screening should begin at 50 years for those individuals at average risk (no family history or genetic syndromes). The ACG endorses colonoscopy as the preferred option. A quality colonoscopy is considered the gold standard for detection and removal of polyps. Other guideline committees feel that a "menu of options" can be employed by both physicians and patients to decide which screening strategy should be used. Colonoscopy as the preferred and gold standard test should be emphasized to patients; however, the other screening options available should also be explained. We believe the ideal screening test and regimen for colon cancer should be individualized. This encompasses taking into account a patient's comorbid illnesses and age and understanding of benefits and risks of the procedure(s) and screening strategies, cost-effectiveness, and availability. We believe it is the physician's responsibility to educate and counsel patients regarding these decisions. Recommended colon cancer screening tests for the average-risk individual starting at age 50 years:

Preferred Test	Alternatives
Colonoscopy every 10 years	FOBT every year
	Flexible sigmoidoscopy every 5 years
	FOBT every year and flexible sigmoidoscopy every 5 years

References

1. Levin B, Lieberman DA, McFarland B, et al; American Cancer Society Colorectal Cancer Advisory Group; US Multi-Society Task Force; American College of Radiology Colon Cancer Committee. Screening and surveillance for the early detection of colorectal cancer and adenomatous polyps, 2008: a joint guideline from the American Cancer Society, the US Multi-Society Task Force on Colorectal Cancer, and the American College of Radiology. *Gastroenterology.* 2008;134(5):1570-1595.

2. US Preventive Services Task Force. Screening for colorectal cancer: U.S Preventive Service Task Force Recommendation Statement. *Annals of Internal Medicine.* 2008;149(9):627-637.

3. Smith RA, Cokkinides V, Eyre HJ. American Cancer Society Guidelines for the Early Detection of Cancer, 2005. *CA Cancer J Clin.* 2005;55(1):31-44; quiz 55-56.

4. Rex DK, Johnson DA, Anderson JC, et al; American College of Gastroenterology. American College of Gastroenterology guidelines for colorectal cancer screening 2009 [corrected]. *Am J Gastroenterol.* 2009;104(3):739-750.

WHAT ARE THE RISK FACTORS FOR COLORECTAL CANCER?

Devina Bhasin, MD and Ashley L. Faulx, MD, FASGE

Colon cancer screening is an important part of our clinical practice. Even when evaluating patients for other medical problems, we discuss proven and potential risk factors for colon cancer and screen patients who have a family history of colorectal cancer (CRC) (Table 38-1).

Nonmodifiable Risk Factors

Age has been shown to be one of the strongest risk factors for the development of colon cancer. The risk of developing colon cancer in the general population is increased with advancing age, with 90% of cancers developing in those age 50 years and older. The prevalence of adenomatous polyps also increases with age and, based on data from the National Polyp Study, so does the risk of having a polyp with high-grade dysplasia.[1]

A family history of colon cancer or adenomatous colon polyps increases the risk for developing colon cancer. In the presence of an affected first-degree relative with colorectal cancer, data from large epidemiologic studies report a relative risk of developing colorectal cancer to be 1.5- to 2-fold greater than that of the general population. Risk is additionally increased if more than one relative is affected and if colorectal cancer was diagnosed prior to age 55. A similar risk also applies if first-degree relatives were found to have adenomatous polyps. For patients with a first-degree relative with colon cancer or adenomatous polyps detected prior to age 50 or for patients with more than one first-degree relative with colon cancer, we typically recommend screening with colonoscopy starting at age 40 or 10 years younger than the earliest diagnosed family member.

Individuals with a personal history of adenomatous polyps or colonic adenocarcinomas are at risk for developing cancer in the future. Adenoma characteristics that are associated with this risk include the presence of 3 or more adenomas, a large (more than 1 cm) adenoma, and polyps with villious or tubulovillious features.[2] In patients who have

---

Table 38-1
Colon Cancer Risk Factors

Known Risk Factors	Possible Risk Factors
Older age	High-fat diet
FAP and variants	High red meat diet
HNPCC and variants	Physical inactivity
Family history of colon cancer	Diabetes mellitus
Personal history of colon cancer/polyps	Radiation exposure
Inflammatory bowel disease	
Cigarette smoking	
Heavy alcohol use	

Adapted from Cappell MS. Pathophysiology, clinical presentation, and management of colon cancer. *Gastroenterol Clin North Am.* 2008;37(1):1-24.

---

had resection for colon cancer, there is an incidence rate of 0.7% for the development of metachronous cancers within the first 2 years postoperatively, warranting close endoscopic surveillance and complete colonic evaluation.[2]

Ulcerative colitis and Crohn's colitis confer an increased risk of colon cancer, primarily though chronic mucosal injury leading to the accumulation of genetic mutations and, ultimately, dysplasia.[3] Patients with ulcerative colitis have a relative risk 2 to 8 times higher than the general population for developing colon cancer. The risk for developing colon cancer correlates most closely with disease duration, beginning about 10 years after the initial diagnosis of pancolitis and 15 to 20 years for left-sided colitis.[4,5] The absolute risk of malignancy increases about 0.5% to 1% yearly after this time, reaching approximately 30% at 35 years for patients with pancolitis. Additionally, several studies suggest that a concurrent diagnosis of primary sclerosing cholangitis along with ulcerative colitis may confer additional risk of for developing colorectal cancer.

Genetic Syndromes Associated With an Increased Risk of Colorectal Cancer

Familial adenomatous polyposis (FAP) results from the germline mutation of the APC gene located on chromosome 5q. Patients with this mutation develop hundreds of colonic adenomas, generally during childhood. Colon cancer occurs in about 90% of individuals by age 45. A variant of FAP, attenuated adenomatous polyposis coli, also has an autosomal dominant mode of inheritance but with fewer adenomas (less than 100) and later age of onset of adenomas and colon cancer. Other variants of FAP include Gardner's syndrome (which has associated osteomas and other extracolonic growths) and Turcot's syndrome (which has a predisposition for colonic polyposis as well as medulloblastomas and other tumors of the central nervous system).

Hereditary nonpolyposis colon cancer (Lynch syndrome) is an autosomal dominant syndrome caused by mutations in DNA mismatch repair genes. Accumulation of mutations within oncogenes and tumor suppressor genes leads to the development of colon cancer at an early age, with particular involvement of the right colon. Colorectal cancer develops in about 80% of individuals with hereditary nonpolyposis coli (HNPCC) at a median age of 48 years. Extracolonic cancers including neoplasms of the stomach, small bowel, ovary, endometrium, and bile duct are also associated with this syndrome. We typically pursue screening colonoscopy in families affected by HNPCC with twice-yearly colonoscopy beginning in the early twenties, then annually after age 40.

Peutz-Jeghers syndrome (PJS) is an autosomal dominant disease characterized by multiple hamartomatous polyps throughout the gastrointestinal tract as well mucocutaneous melanin deposition involving the lips, buccal mucosa, hands, and feet.[6] Patients with PJS have a 39% estimated lifetime risk of developing colon cancer, primarily due to the development of adenomatous tissue within the hamartomatous polyps.

Juvenile polyposis is an autosomal dominant condition associated with an increased risk of colorectal cancer. Individuals with juvenile polyposis have a family history of gastrointestinal malignancy and multiple juvenile polyps that may arise from the colon, stomach, and small intestine. Juvenile polyposis is often associated with cardiac and congenital abnormalities as well.[2]

Lifestyle and Exposures Associated With an Increased Colorectal Cancer Risk

Lifestyle and other factors that have been implicated in increasing risk of colorectal cancer include diet, alcohol use, cigarette smoking, physical inactivity, and diabetes. Diets high in red or processed meat have been shown to be associated with increased risk of colorectal cancer based on several case-control studies in the United States and Europe, though prospective studies of low-fat, high-fiber diets have been inconclusive. The relative risk of colon cancer and high intake of red and processed meat is approximately 1.41.[7] Several studies have suggested an increase in colon cancer risk from between 10% and 25% in those with excessive daily alcohol consumption. Cigarette smoking, based on several meta-analyses of prospective studies, observational studies, and cohort studies, has also been associated with increased incidence of colon cancer with an approximate relative risk of 1.2 compared with nonsmokers. In several studies using different measures of activity, sedentary individuals had twice the incidence of colon cancer compared with those who had a high level of activity. A possible basis for this association is that, in general, exercise stimulates intestinal peristalsis and thus reduces mucosal contact with carcinogens while stimulating immunosurveillance. Diabetes mellitus has also been linked with an increased risk of colon cancer, possibly due to insulin-induced colonic mucosal and tumor cell proliferation. A meta-analysis found that those with diabetes had an approximately 30% increased risk of colon cancer compared with nondiabetics.[8] We typically do not adjust standard screening practice for the above lifestyle factors at this time, though this may change with future research in this field.

Lastly, prior abdominal or pelvic radiation exposure, generally in the form of prior radiation therapy to treat malignancy, may increase the risk of developing CRC. Individuals with a history of bladder, prostate, or gynecologic malignancies should be queried regarding prior radiation exposure and possibly screened more often and starting from a younger age.

References

1. Winawer SJ, Zauber AG, Gerdes H, et al. Risk of colorectal cancer in the families of patients with adenomatous polyps. National Polyp Study Workgroup. *N Engl J Med.* 1996;334(2):82-87.
2. Kastrinos F, Syngal S. Colorectal cancer screening. In: Greenberger NJ, Blumberg RS, eds. *Current Diagnosis and Treatment: Gastroenterology, Hepatology, and Endoscopy.* New York, NY: McGraw Hill Companies; 2009:257-278.
3. Cappell MS. Pathophysiology, clinical presentation, and management of colon cancer. *Gastroenterol Clin North Am.* 2008;37(1):1-24.
4. Greenstein AJ, Sachar DB, Smith H, et al. Cancer in universal and left-sided colitis: factors determining risk. *Gastroenterology.* 1979;77(2):290-294.
5. Ekbom A, Helmick C, Zack M, Adami HO. Ulcerative colitis and colorectal cancer. A population based study. *N Engl J Med.* 1990;323(18):1228-1233.
6. Bresalier R, Kim Y. Malignant neoplasms of the large intestine. In: Feldman M, Scharschmidt BF, eds. *Sleisenger & Fordtran's Gastrointestinal and Liver Disease.* 6th ed. Philadelphia, PA: WB Saunders Company; 1998: 1907-1919.
7. Chao A, Thun MJ, Connell CJ, et al. Meat consumption and risk of colorectal cancer. *JAMA.* 2005;293(2): 172-182.
8. Larsson SC, Orsini N, Wolk A. Diabetes mellitus and risk of colorectal cancer: a meta-analysis. *J Natl Cancer Inst.* 2005;97(22):1679-1687.
9. Thun MJ, Calle EE, Namboodiri MM, et al. Risk factors for fatal colon cancer in a large prospective study. *J Natl Cancer Inst.* 1992;84(19):1491-1500.

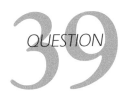

WHAT SURGICAL OPTIONS ARE AVAILABLE FOR PATIENTS WITH COLON CANCER, INCLUDING THOSE WHO PRESENT WITH ACUTE OBSTRUCTION?

Clifford S. Cho, MD, FACS

Despite considerable improvements in chemotherapy, surgical resection remains the only potentially curative intervention for patients with colon adenocarcinoma. However, the ways in which surgical resection can be delivered are varied. This chapter will describe how to best tailor the nature and timing of operative intervention to the clinical circumstance at hand.

The optimal mode of surgical treatment is determined by the nature of the clinical presentation. The ways in which colon adenocarcinoma can manifest itself are variable, but for purposes of surgical decision making, you may categorize a patient's clinical presentation with 3 questions:

1. Where is the primary tumor (or tumors)?

2. Does the patient have metastatic disease?

3. Is the patient unstable (in need of urgent operative intervention)?

The first question is usually answered by endoscopic colonoscopy or computed tomography (CT) scan. The second question is answered by radiographic studies such as computed tomographic imaging. Ideally, all 3 questions should be answered prior to embarking on an operative intervention. However, if the answer to the third question is "yes," the luxury of complete oncologic staging may not be available.

The type of resection to perform depends on the anatomic location of the primary tumor, but the operative conduct of each procedure is motivated by 3 goals: local control, nodal staging, and construction of a tension-free intestinal anastomosis.

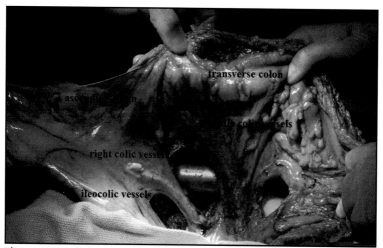

Figure 39-1. Intraoperative photograph demonstrating the vessels that are ligated and the portions of colon that are resected in an extended right hemicolectomy.

Optimization of local control (that is, prevention of local tumor recurrence) requires that the tumor be resected with widely negative margins. The redundancy of the colon generally makes it quite easy to resect colonic tumors with 5-cm margins. Recent analyses have suggested that optimal nodal staging requires that at least 12 lymph nodes be examined in order to accurately distinguish stage II (node-negative) from stage III (node-positive) cases.[1] To accomplish this, a broad segment of mesentery adjacent to the resected segment of colon must also be removed. Because the nodal drainage of the colon runs along its vascular inflow, this requires that the arterial inflow of the resected colonic segment be divided at its point of origin off the aorta. Finally, to avoid anastomotic leakage, it is of utmost importance that the intestinal anastomosis be constructed in a way that minimizes tension. This requires extensive operative mobilization of the segments of small intestine or colon to be reconnected.

To accomplish these 3 goals, tumors of the cecum and ascending colon are resected with a *right hemicolectomy,* in which the right colon and the nodal tissue along the ileocolic and right colic arteries are harvested, and an ileocolic anastomosis is constructed between the distal ileum and proximal transverse colon. Tumors of the proximal-to-middle transverse colon occasionally require an *extended right hemicolectomy,* in which the right colon and proximal transverse colon are resected along with the nodal basin along the ileocolic, right, and middle colic arteries (Figure 39-1). On occasion, tumors of the mid-transverse colon may be resected with a *transverse colectomy,* in which the transverse colon and the nodal basin along the middle colic artery are resected. In this operation, the peritoneal attachments of the ascending colon and descending colon must be mobilized in order to construct a tension-free anastomosis between them. Tumors of the middle-to-distal transverse colon may occasionally require an *extended left hemicolectomy,* in which the distal transverse colon and descending colon are resected with the nodal basin along the middle and left colic arteries. Tumors of the descending colon are resected with a *left hemicolectomy* that includes the nodal basis along the left colic artery, and tumors of the sigmoid colon can be resected with a *sigmoid colectomy* (also referred to as an *anterior resection*), in which the redundant sigmoid colon is resected with the lymph nodes along the sigmoid artery, and the descending colon is anastomosed to the proximal rectum. On occasion, patients with multiple tumors may require a *subtotal colectomy*, which encompasses all of these operations.

For each of these operative procedures, the oncologic equivalence between open and laparoscopic colectomy has been established.[2,3] As a result, laparoscopic colectomies are currently being performed in a growing plurality of cases.

In the presence of stage IV (metastatic) disease, I generally try to avoid surgical resection of the primary tumor as the initial therapeutic intervention. In stage IV colon adenocarcinoma, the primary determinants of long-term outcome are distant metastases and not the primary colonic tumor. Thanks to the considerable advancements that have been made in systemic chemotherapy during the past decade, the median survival of patients with even inoperable and widely metastatic colon adenocarcinoma currently exceeds 2 years. For patients with stage IV disease whose primary colon tumors are asymptomatic, the likelihood of developing complications caused by progression of the primary tumor (such as colonic obstruction or bleeding) during administration of systemic chemotherapy is very low.[4] Therefore, these patients are usually best served by providing them with the treatment they need most: systemic chemotherapy. Early operative intervention will only delay their receipt of this treatment. A large subset of these patients may ultimately be candidates for potentially curative surgical therapy (such as colectomy and partial hepatectomy to resect their synchronous liver metastases). In these patients, a course of systemic chemotherapy allows for a period of observation during which the possible onset of additional foci of disease can be monitored and the *in vivo* responsiveness of their disease to chemotherapy can be assessed. After this period of observation, patients who are determined to have surgically resectable disease are offered colectomy and metastasectomy. In young or healthy patients, I try to perform these operative procedures concurrently.

The ability to optimally evaluate a primary colon cancer and the possibility of metastatic disease can be limited when complications resulting from the primary colonic tumor are present. These include obstruction, hemorrhage, and/or colonic perforation. Whenever possible, one should try to manage acute complications nonoperatively. Nonoperative management may provide enough time to collect the answers to Questions 1 and 2 (see p. 197) that may allow you to select the most appropriate surgical option.

For patients presenting with obstruction, endoscopic insertion of a self-expanding colonic stent generally results in colonic decompression allowing for colonoscopy or CT scanning to exclude synchronous colonic lesions and cross-sectional imaging to exclude synchronous extraintestinal metastases. For patients with significant hemorrhage, angiographic embolization will identify the anatomic location of the bleeding tumor and may stabilize the patient long enough to undertake appropriate preoperative staging evaluations. For clinically stable patients presenting with a contained colonic perforation, initiation of antimicrobial therapy and percutaneous drainage of the resulting abscess allows for appropriate diagnostic testing prior to operation.

Operative intervention must be undertaken immediately for patients with obstruction or bleeding that is not amenable to nonoperative maneuvers regardless of tumor stage, as well as for patients with free colonic perforation resulting in diffuse peritonitis.

Several important considerations for patients presenting with perforation deserve attention. One circumstance to consider is when perforation results in significant peritoneal soiling. Under these conditions, the risk of anastomotic failure is quite high, so no attempt at intestinal anastomosis should be undertaken. Internal anastomosis is also difficult to accomplish in patients with acute obstruction who have not undergone preoperative bowel preparation. In these patients, a diverting stoma is constructed, which may be reversed at a later date after completion of postoperative healing and possible adjuvant chemotherapy. Another element to consider is that obstructing colon cancers are usually found in the left colon; moreover, they generally do not result in perforation at the site of tumor, but at the cecum. As a result, operative resection of the obstructing tumor and the site of perforation often requires a subtotal colectomy with diverting ileostomy. Although colonic perforation places patients at higher risk of disease recurrence, the outcomes after resection are not uniformly poor; therefore, whenever possible, effort should be expended to perform an oncologically appropriate resection. Obviously, if a patient is hemodynamically unstable at the time of operation, an abbreviated resection may become necessary. In these circumstances, a limited resection of the affected segment of colon with a proximally diverting ostomy may suffice.

References

1. Nelson H, Petrelli N, Carlin A, et al. Guidelines 2000 for colon and rectal cancer surgery. *J Natl Clin Inst.* 2001;93(8):583-596.
2. Fleshman J, Sargent DJ, Green E, et al. Laparoscopic colectomy for cancer is not inferior to open surgery based on 5-year data from the COST study group. *Ann Surg.* 2007;246(3):655-662.
3. Kennedy GD, Heise C, Rajamanickam V, et al. Laparoscopy decreases postoperative complication rates after abdominal colectomy: results from the national surgical quality improvement program. *Ann Surg.* 2009;249(4):596-601.
4. Poultsides GA, Servais EL, Saltz LB, et al. Outcome of primary tumor in patients with synchronous stage IV colorectal cancer receiving combination chemotherapy without surgery as initial treatment. *J Clin Oncol.* 2009;27(20):3379-3384.

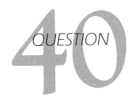

How Should Patients With a Solitary Liver Metastasis From Colon Cancer Be Evaluated and Treated?

Clifford S. Cho, MD, FACS

Improvements in chemotherapy, operative, and perioperative management have revolutionized the treatment of patients with hepatic metastases from colorectal adenocarcinoma. Favorable long-term survival outcomes can now be expected for a plurality of patients presenting with solitary liver metastases from colon cancer. However, the key to success when treating these patients is to understand how to best coordinate the use of medical and surgical oncologic therapies.

Proper evaluation of liver metastases requires some familiarity with basic hepatic anatomy. The liver can be subdivided into 2 hemilivers (right and left) or 8 anatomic segments (segments I through VIII). The right hemiliver (segments V through VIII) and left hemiliver (segments II through IV) are anatomically divided by the middle hepatic vein, which runs between the two. The right hemiliver is further subdivided into the right anterior section (segments V and VIII) and right posterior section (segments VI and VII); these are anatomically divided by the right hepatic vein, which runs between the two. Segment IV of the left hemiliver is visually separable from segments II and III by the umbilical fissure, which runs between them. The caudate lobe, or segment I, is situated between the right and left hemilivers and resides in a space between the portal vein and inferior vena cava.

Hepatic tissue is perfused dually from the portal venous and hepatic arterial systems. The majority of hepatocellular perfusion is delivered through the portal vein, which enters the hepatic hilus at the porta hepatic and divides into the right and left portal veins. In general, the right portal vein enters the liver parenchyma where it bifurcates into a right anterior sectional pedicle that perfuses the right anterior section of the liver (segments V and VIII) and a right posterior sectional pedicle that perfuses the right posterior section of the liver (segments VI and VII). In contrast, the left portal vein typically runs obliquely outside the liver parenchyma and enters the umbilical fissure to give rise to branches that perfuse segments II, III, and IV. The caudate lobe (segment I) derives its blood supply from both the right and left portal veins. The hepatic arterial system generally follows a similar anatomic pattern. In contrast, hepatobiliary anatomy is highly prone to variation, and operative therapy demands a close familiarity with common anatomic variants.

Venous outflow from the liver is conducted into the right, middle, and left hepatic veins. As stated, the right hepatic vein runs between the right anterior and right posterior sections and drains blood from both. The middle hepatic vein runs between the right anterior section and segment IV of the left hemiliver and drains blood from both. The left hepatic vein runs between segments II and III of the left hemiliver and drains blood from both. All 3 veins enter the inferior vena cava above the liver, with the left and middle veins usually forming a short common trunk prior to entering the vena cava.

The best way to begin the evaluation and treatment of patients with solitary liver metastases from colon cancer is to determine their operative resectability. The ability to resect tumors from the liver is facilitated by the unique capacity of the liver to regenerate after partial hepatectomy. In healthy patients, up to 80% of the liver may be safely removed, with the expectation that the remaining liver will be capable of sufficient hypertrophy to eventually restore normal hepatic function. Resection of too much liver tissue, or significant compromise to the health of the remaining portion of liver, can result in postoperative hepatic insufficiency that is often fatal. Understanding these limits of operative intervention is the key to determining resectability; this determination is made not by evaluating the portion of the liver that is to be removed, but by calculating the portion of the liver that will be left behind. Specifically, 3 anatomic variables must be considered to determine a patient's candidacy for operative resection: inflow, outflow, and volume.

In order for the future liver remnant to be capable of sustaining enough hypertrophy to maintain adequate liver function, the portal vein and hepatic artery perfusing that portion of liver must remain intact following operative resection. Thus, if a tumor involves a portion of the vascular inflow to the intended liver remnant, it must be considered unresectable (Figure 40-1). Similarly, hepatic venous outflow must be retained in order for a liver remnant to survive. Therefore, if a tumor involves a portion of the vascular outflow from the intended liver remnant, it must be considered unresectable (Figure 40-2). Finally, there is a minimum volume of liver that must be retained in order to permit its survival. In general, a safe minimum requirement is to leave at least 25% of the total liver volume intact following resection. However, for patients with underlying liver dysfunction from steatosis, fibrosis, cirrhosis, or chemotherapy-induced hepatotoxicity, the minimum volume may be between 30% and 40%. Hepatic volumes can be calculated using software based on standard computed tomography. If resection of a tumor will result in a future liver remnant whose volume is smaller than the minimum volume required, it must be considered unresectable.

If a patient is found to be resectable, one must decide when to undertake operative intervention. Some authors have advocated the use of neoadjuvant systemic chemotherapy for patients with resectable hepatic metastases. One rationale for this is that these patients with stage IV colon cancer will eventually require systemic treatment, and the presence of a radiographically evaluable tumor in the liver can serve as an *in vivo* means of testing the sensitivity of a patient's cancer to chemotherapy (by observing tumor regression). A caveat to this is the phenomenon of chemotherapy-induced hepatotoxicity; sustained use of contemporary chemotherapy agents has been shown to induce hepatic steatosis and sinusoidal obstruction that can increase the risk of resection and weaken the ability of the liver to hypertrophy following resection.[1] In my practice, I favor proceeding toward

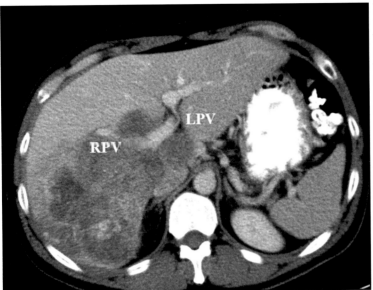

Figure 40-1. A 51-year-old man initially presented with a right-sided liver metastases involving both the right portal vein (RPV) and left portal vein (LPV), rendering his tumor technically unresectable.

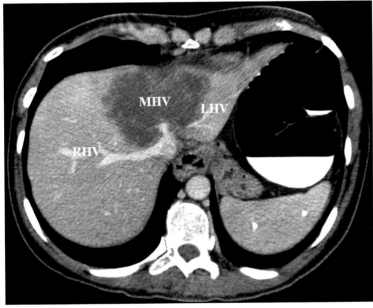

Figure 40-2. A 50-year-old woman initially presented with a centrally located liver metastasis that involved the left hepatic vein (LHV), middle hepatic vein (MHV), and right hepatic vein (RHV), rendering her tumor technically unresectable.

operative resection without neoadjuvant chemotherapy for patients with resectable hepatic metastases. However, this controversy is the subject of ongoing prospective studies.

If a patient is found to be technically unresectable due to inadequate inflow, outflow, or volume of the anticipated future liver remnant, adjunctive therapy should be considered. Contemporary systemic chemotherapy is highly effective at producing regression of hepatic colorectal metastases and has been shown to be capable of converting a subset of unresectable patients to resectability. This can be achieved by inducing local regression of tumor away from critical vascular structures that may permit adequate inflow or outflow to the anticipated future liver remnant (Figure 40-3). Another adjunct to consider is portal vein embolization, which is a means of increasing the size of the anticipated future liver

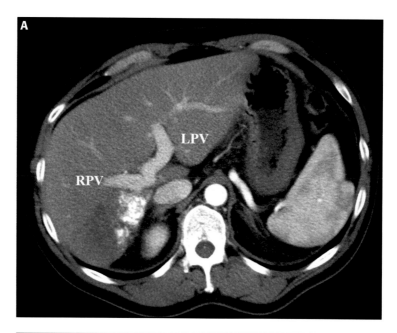

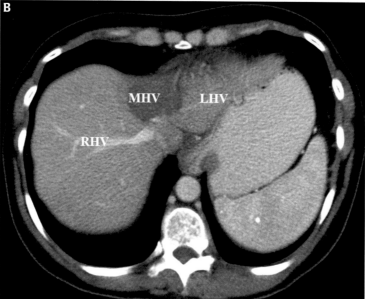

Figure 40-3. (A) Following systemic chemotherapy, the right-sided lesion present in the 51-year-old man described in Figure 40-1 regressed to the point of involving only the right portal vein, making him eligible for resection in the form of an extended right hemihepatectomy. (B) Following systemic chemotherapy, the centrally located lesion present in the 50-year-old woman described in Figure 40-2 regressed to the point of involving only the left and middle hepatic veins, permitting resection in the form of an extended left hemihepatectomy.

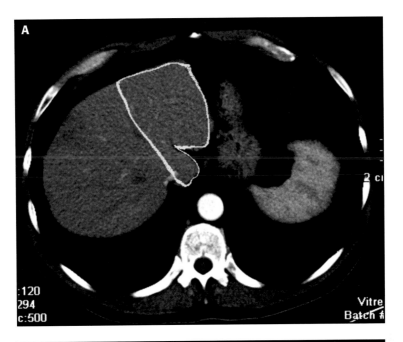

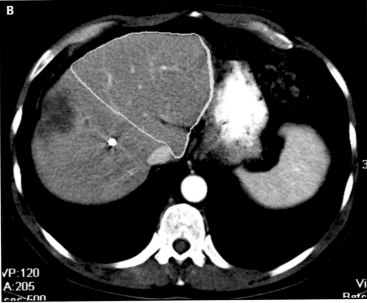

Figure 40-4. (A) A 63-year-old man with right-sided hepatic rectal adenocarcinoma metastases treated with systemic chemotherapy initially presented with an estimated future liver remnant volume of 23%. (B) Following right portal vein embolization, the estimated future liver remnant volume increased to 36%, permitting resection in the form of a right hemihepatectomy.

remnant. By inducing ipsilateral atrophy and contralateral hypertrophy, embolization of the portal vein supplying the portion of the liver to be resected can effectively increase the size of the future liver remnant and appears to increase the tolerability of extended hepatic resections (Figure 40-4).[2,3] Therefore, close and serial radiographic follow-up should be undertaken for all patients with technically unresectable hepatic disease over the course of chemotherapy.

A growing number of centers are performing even major hepatectomies laparoscopically.[4] Early analyses suggest that perioperative outcomes may be favorable with this approach. Another treatment modality to consider, particularly for patients with relatively small tumors and medical comorbidities that may not permit hepatic resection, is tumor ablation. Percutaneous, laparoscopic, or open radiofrequency, microwave, or cryoablation has been shown to be effective in local control of tumors, and ongoing technological improvements are likely to broaden the indications and efficacy of these interventions. However, it remains to be determined if ablative techniques have yet achieved the oncologic outcomes associated with formal hepatic resection.

References

1. Karoui M, Penna C, Amin-Hashem M, et al. Influence of preoperative chemotherapy on the risk of major hepatectomy for colorectal liver metastases. *Ann Surg.* 2006;243(1):1-7.
2. Riberto D, Abdalla EK, Madoff DC, et al. Portal vein embolization before major hepatectomy and its effects on regeneration, resectability, and outcome. *Br J Surg.* 2007;94(11):1386-1394.
3. Wicherts DA, Miller R, de Haas RJ, et al. Long-term results of two-stage hepatectomy for irresectable colorectal cancer liver metastases. *Ann Surg.* 2008;248(6):994-1005.
4. Kazaryan AM, Pavlik Marangos I, Rosseland AR, et al. Laparoscopic liver resection for malignant and benign lesions: ten-year Norwegian single center experience. *Arch Surg.* 2010;145(1):34-40.

41

WHICH PATIENTS WITH COLORECTAL CANCER SHOULD BE CONSIDERED FOR A COLONIC STENT?

Jeffrey Laczek, MD and Peter Darwin, MD

Of the 148,000 patients in the United States who develop colorectal cancer annually, a substantial number will present with or develop colonic obstruction. Colonic obstruction had historically been addressed via surgical approaches, with acute colonic obstruction requiring emergency intervention and patients with chronic obstructive symptoms requiring elective surgical procedures.

The introduction into clinical practice of colonic stents in the 1990s opened the door for the endoscopic treatment of colonic obstruction. In patients with colonic obstruction, the stent may either serve as a bridge to surgery or as a definitive palliative treatment.

Patients who present with an acute colonic obstruction are at risk for bowel perforation with accompanying sepsis and require urgent decompression; acute colonic obstruction thus represents a medical/surgical emergency. The presenting signs and symptoms may include abdominal pain, nausea and vomiting (sometimes with feculent emesis), abdominal distension, and the inability to pass stool or flatus. While a standard abdominal X-ray series (KUB and upright films) may demonstrate an obstructed bowel gas pattern, computed tomography (CT) imaging with water-soluble oral and intravenous (IV) contrast better delineates the precise location of the lesion and the presence or absence of gross metastatic disease.

The standard surgical management of such patients requires resection with possible colostomy. Primary colo-colonic anastomosis is often not possible in these patients as they have not undergone a standard bowel preparation prior to surgery. When the patient is more stable and after recovering from the acute surgery, a second surgery for ostomy "takedown" and the creation of an internal anastomosis can be performed.

To avoid a 2-stage operation, temporary, preoperative stent placement has been widely used as a bridge to an elective resection. A colonic stent allows bowel decompression, formal bowel preparation, and optimization of comorbid conditions prior to an elective

Figure 41-1. Endoscopic view of wire placement across malignant colon obstruction.

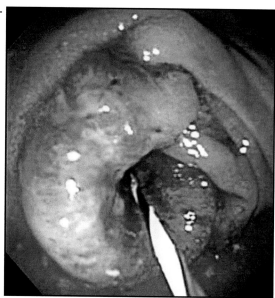

Figure 41-2. Endoscopic view of colon stent immediately after deployment.

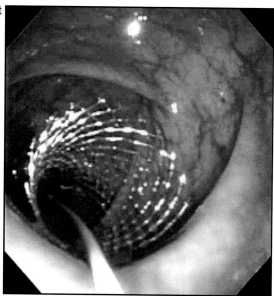

resection with the intent of creating a primary re-anastomosis. Rectal cancers are often treated with neoadjuvant chemotherapy and radiation prior to resection, further arguing for colonic stenting and against urgent surgical intervention.

We advocate considering colonic stents as a bridge to surgery in all patients with complete or clinically significant colonic obstruction, particularly in those who would benefit from the stabilization of comorbid diseases (Figures 41-1 and 41-2).

The use of stents for definitive palliation in patients who have advanced/unresectable disease or who are poor surgical candidates with incomplete/high-grade obstruction is also widely performed and in many centers is the mainstay of care. Colonic stent placement has a low mortality rate (less than 1%) but is associated with a higher rate of long-term complications than surgery, mostly due to stent-related complications (such as repeat

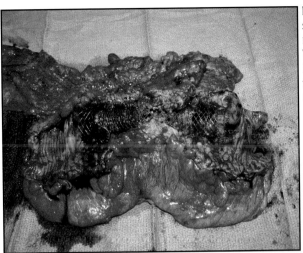

Figure 41-3. Pathologic specimen consisting of a primary colon cancer surrounding a previously placed colonic Wallflex stent (Boston Scientific, Natick, Massachusetts) removed *en bloc* at the time of surgery. (Reprinted with permission of Douglas G. Adler, MD.)

obstruction due to tumor ingrowth or overgrowth through the stent wall interstices). In one large meta-analysis, complications of stent placement were perforation (3.8%), stent migration (11.8%), and re-obstruction (7.3%).[1] Most patients with stent obstruction due to tumor overgrowth/ingrowth can be managed via tumor debridement via argon plasma coagulation or, more commonly, via the placement of a second stent inside the first one (so-called "stent-within-stent" deployment). Stent placement should be considered in patients who have advanced co-morbidities or anatomic considerations (ie, dense adhesions) that make them high-risk operative candidates. Stents are likewise useful in patients who have other reasons to delay surgery (family events, etc) but these are less commonly encountered.

It should be noted that a patient's overall clinical situation and tumor stage may not be available or may not be clear at the time of presentation with acute colonic obstruction (ie, a CT may not have been performed with IV contrast, imaging may be limited due to inability of the patient to take oral contrast, etc). In such cases, it is reasonable to empirically place a colonic stent and allow colonic decompression and patient stabilization. When the patient is more stable clinically and full staging can be performed, a decision can be made about whether or not the stent should be removed *en bloc* with tumor at the time of surgery or left in place as a palliative measure if the patient is found to have advanced or unresectable disease (Figure 41-3).

As stool remains primarily liquid in the right colon, high-grade bowel obstruction due to proximal colon cancers is less commonly encountered. Our general practice is to avoid stent placement in these patients unless there are significant obstructive symptoms, in which case stents can be placed. Several large case series have demonstrated that proximal colonic stenting is safe and effective with clinical outcomes similar to those seen for distal tumors.[2]

For lesions of the rectosigmoid colon, formed stool in conjunction with a high-grade stenosis may cause obstruction, and some form of treatment in short order should be considered. Stool softeners and maintenance of adequate hydration can be used while awaiting resection or neoadjuvant therapy. If surgery is not feasible, long-term stenting of the rectosigmoid can be performed either for a high-grade or complete obstruction.

There are several other factors to consider in patients being considered for colon stents. First, patients with clinical or radiologic evidence of peritonitis, perforation, or significant gastrointestinal bleeding are not candidates for colonic stenting and should undergo surgical therapy. Second, patients with a shorter length of obstruction (ie, 6 cm or less) do better after colon stent placement than patients with longer obstructions.[3] Treatment of very distal obstructions in the rectum (less than 5 cm from the anal verge) has been reported, but must be balanced against the risks of incontinence and patient discomfort, although it is difficult to predict which patients will develop these complications.[4] Some patients will accept these risks in order to avoid an ostomy.

Patients with extrinsic colonic obstruction, most commonly due to advanced gynecologic cancers, can also be considered for colonic stenting. These patients are often poor surgical candidates with short life expectancies and few therapeutic options available. Colonic stents placed in this situation have a higher risk of migration as they are being placed up against largely normal, albeit compressed, colonic tissue. Colonic strictures in these patients tend to be longer than in those with primary colorectal cancers, and in some cases overlapping stents may be required to bridge an obstruction. Colonic stents work well in this admittedly difficult clinical setting.

In any situation where a colonic stent is used, close communication between the gastroenterologist, surgeon, and patient is required. We are strong proponents of the use of colonic stents as a bridge to surgery in patients presenting with obstructing colon cancer, as this is associated with a higher rate of 1-step surgical resection and allows time to optimize comorbid conditions. A 1-step surgery obviates a colostomy, improving patients' quality of life. As a definite therapy, we generally reserve colonic stents for patients who have a high perioperative risk or for patients with a short life expectancy. When stents are used as definitive palliation, patients need to be aware of the long-term complications, such as perforation (including delayed perforation), migration, and re-obstruction.

References

1. Sevastian S, Johnston S, Geoghegan T, Torreggiani W, Buckley M. Pooled analysis of the efficacy and safety of self-expanding metal stenting in malignant colo-rectal obstruction. *Am J Gastroenterol.* 2004;99(10): 2051-2057.
2. Repici A, Adler D, Gibbs CM, Malesci A, Preatoni P, Baron TH. Stenting the proximal colon in patients with malignant large bowel obstruction: techniques and outcomes. *Gastrointest Endosc.* 2007;66(5):940-944.
3. Jung MK, Park SY, Jeon SW, et al. Factors associated with the long-term outcome of a self-expandable colon stent used for palliation of malignant colorectal obstruction. *Surg Endosc.* 2010;24(3):525-530.
4. Song HY, Kim JH, Kim KR, et al. Malignant rectal obstruction within 5 cm of the anal verge: is there a role for expandable metallic stent placement? *Gastrointest Endosc.* 2008;68(4):713-720.

What Is the Best Surveillance Regimen for Patients Following Colon Cancer Resection?

David Chu, MD and Douglas G. Adler, MD, FACG, AGAF, FASGE

Colorectal cancer recurrence following curative surgical resection is a major concern. Tumor may manifest as local recurrence or via the formation of new, metachronous tumors. Despite current colorectal cancer treatment regimens, the overall recurrence rate remains significant (16% to 33%).[1-3] Local recurrence occurs significantly more often in rectal cancers than in colon cancers, and outcomes for both are generally improved with surgery (5-year survival rate 47.7%) compared to without (10.3%).[1] The rate of anastomotic recurrence is low and is usually associated with advanced intra-abdominal and pelvic invasive disease. Postresection surveillance for local recurrence alone is considered low-yield, and studies have not shown a significant mortality benefit, arguing for more global post-treatment surveillance.[4]

The risk of developing metachronous tumors is genetically based and significantly elevated (lifetime risk 33%) in an individual who has already developed a primary colon cancer.[5] Surgical resection and chemoradiotherapy for the initial tumor do not prevent the occurrence of a secondary, metachronous tumor (Figure 42-1).[6]

Current surveillance guidelines are designed to detect these secondary cancers at an early stage to allow for curative endoscopic or, more commonly, surgical resection. In general, noninvasive tests used for the primary prevention of colorectal cancer (fecal occult blood testing, fecal immunochemical testing, and stool DNA testing) are not indicated for surveillance in this high-risk population.[6,7] Current guidelines recommend direct visualization of any remaining colon via colonoscopy as the test of choice.[4,8]

Figure 42-1. Metachronous cecal cancer detected on colonoscopy 3 years after resection of a sigmoid colon cancer. CT revealed no evidence of spread, and the patient underwent curative resection.

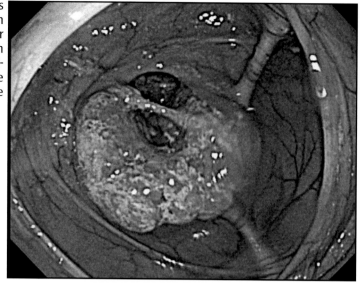

Role of Colonoscopy

The mean yield of surveillance colonoscopy in postresection patients has been reported to be 17.2% for adenomatous polyps and 7.6% for colon cancer.[9] Detection of recurrence via colonoscopy was reported to have a mortality benefit in several studies; however, this benefit did not always reach statistical significance.[10,11] Approximately one metachronous cancer is detected per 157 colonoscopies in patients with a history of colorectal cancer.[12] The majority of metachronous cancers (65%) are considered surgically resectable at the time of diagnosis.[4]

Current guidelines recommend that patients with known colorectal cancer undergo complete colon evaluation to rule out synchronous lesions. In nonobstructive tumors, preoperative colonoscopy is performed. In patients with obstructive tumors in whom complete colonoscopy cannot be performed, computed tomography (CT) colonography or double-contrast barium enema should be performed to evaluate for the presence of any other tumors in the colon. In patients who undergo radiographic studies only, in the absence of unresectable metastatic disease, it is suggested that colonoscopy be performed 3 to 6 months after surgery to rule out synchronous disease.

All disease-free individuals with any remaining large bowel should receive colonoscopy 1-year postresection. If negative, this should be followed up by repeat colonoscopy in 3 years and again in 5 years.[4] The majority of recurrences occur within 2 years postresection, and screening is not recommended past the 5-year interval or in individuals who have less than 10 years of life expectancy.[4,13]

Colonoscopies are heavily dependent on the quality of the bowel preparation at the time of the exam. If a suboptimal study is obtained, then a follow-up colonoscopy should be performed in a timely fashion. In addition, there may be an emotional component of reassurance in colorectal cancer survivors that warrants more frequent screening intervals or extended periods of screening. Ordering colonoscopies should be left to the clinician's discretion in these cases.

Role of Carcinoembryonic Antigen Monitoring

As of now, carcinoembryonic antigen (CEA) is the only tumor marker recommended for postresection surveillance of colorectal cancer. The overall sensitivity and specificity for detecting colon cancer recurrence are 64% and 90%, respectively. A CEA level of 2.2 ng/mL was suggested as a cut-off point to balance sensitivity and specificity.[14] The most recent guidelines suggest CEA monitoring every 3 months for a total of 3 years in individuals with stage II or III cancers who would be candidates for curative surgery or chemotherapy. Elevated CEA levels should warrant additional workup for recurrent disease. CEA levels can be elevated postchemotherapy, and those levels should be interpreted with caution.[15]

Role of Imaging

The utility of imaging in surveillance for recurrent colorectal cancer is unclear. Double-contrast barium enema (DCBE) is less sensitive than colonoscopy in detecting recurrence postpolypectomy and is not recommended to detect recurrence postsurgical resection.[16] In primary screening, CT colonography is comparable to colonoscopy for lesions 10 mm or smaller, but is less sensitive for smaller lesions.[17] The role of CT colonography in the setting of recurrence remains unclear at this time, but it can detect extracolonic findings.[7]

PET-CT has not been extensively studied in the detection of recurrence in postresection patients. In the detection of primary cancers, PET-CT was shown to have a sensitivity of 52% and specificity of 93%. However, PET-CT failed to detect significant colonic findings in 11.8% of cases, including 5% of colon cancers and lymphomas, and does not replace the role of colonoscopy.[18] PET-CT may have false-negative results in tumors with low metabolic activity.[19] There may be an intermediate role in using PET-CT to follow-up abnormal CEA levels and pursuing colonoscopy if significant pathology is detected.[8]

Conclusion

Recurrence of colorectal cancer postcurative resection can be a cause of significant mortality and morbidity. Current guidelines recommend colonoscopy as the initial step in asymptomatic patients with regular follow-up at 1, 3, and 5 years postresection. CEA levels should be followed as per guidelines and investigated if elevated. At this time, other surveillance modalities are considered either adjuncts to colonoscopy or are not recommended outside of research protocols.

References

1. Yun HR, Lee LJ, Cho YK, et al. Local recurrence after curative resection in patients with colon and rectal cancers. *Int J Colorectal Dis.* 2008;23(11):1081-1087.
2. O'Connell MJ, Campbell ME, Goldberg RM, et al. Survival following recurrence in stage II and III colon cancer: findings from the ACCENT data set. *J Clin Oncol.* 2008;26(14):2336-2341.
3. Kobayashi H, Mochizuki H, Morita T, et al. Timing of relapse and outcome after curative resection for colorectal cancer: a Japanese multicenter study. *Dig Surg.* 2009;26(3):249-255.
4. Brooks DD, Winawer SJ, Rex DK, et al; Postsurgical Surveillance of Colorectal Cancer Study Group, Japanese Society for Cancer of the Colon and Rectum. Colonoscopy surveillance after polypectomy and colorectal cancer resection. *Am Fam Physician.* 2008;77(7):995-1004.

5. Grady WM, Carethers JM. Genomic and epigenetic instability in colorectal cancer pathogenesis. *Gastroenterology.* 2008;135(4):1079-1099.

6. Carethers JM. Secondary prevention of colorectal cancer: is there an optimal follow-up for patients with colorectal cancer? *Curr Colorectal Cancer Rep.* 2010;6(1):24-29.

7. Levin B, Lieberman DA, McFarland B, et al; American Cancer Society Colorectal Cancer Advisory Group, US Multi-Society Task Force, American College of Radiology Colon Cancer Committee. Screening and surveillance for the early detection of colorectal cancer and adenomatous polyps, 2008: a joint guideline from the American Cancer Society, the US Multi-Society Task Force on Colorectal Cancer, and the American College of Radiology. *CA Cancer J Clin.* 2008;58(3):130-160.

8. Arditi C, Gonvers JJ, Burnand B, et al; EPAGE II Study Group. Appropriateness of colonoscopy in Europe (EPAGE II) surveillance after polypectomy and after resection of colorectal cancer. *Endoscopy.* 2009;41(3): 209-217.

9. Froehlich F, Gonvers JJ. Diagnostic yield of colonoscopy by indication. In: Waye JD, Rex DK, Williams CB (eds). *Colonoscopy: Principles and Practice.* Oxford: Blackwell Publishing; 2003:111.

10. Rodriguez-Moranta F, Salo J, Arcusa A, et al. Postoperative surveillance in patients with colorectal cancer who have undergone curative resection: a prospective, multicenter, randomized, controlled trial. *J Clin Oncol.* 2006;24(3):386-393.

11. Secco GB, Fardelli R, Gianquinto D, et al. Efficacy and cost of risk-adapted follow-up in patients after colorectal cancer surgery: a prospective, randomized and controlled trial. *Eur J Surg Oncol.* 2002;28(4):418-423.

12. Langevin JM, Nivatvongs S. The true incidence of synchronous cancer of the large bowel. A prospective study. *Am J Surg.* 1984;147(3):330-333.

13. Green RJ, Metlay JP, Propert K, et al. Surveillance for second primary colorectal cancer after adjuvant chemotherapy: an analysis of Intergroup 0089. *Ann Intern Med.* 2002;136(4):261-269.

14. Tan E, Gouvas N, Nicholls RJ, et al. Diagnostic precision of carcinoembryonic antigen in the detection of recurrence of colorectal cancer. *Surg Oncol.* 2009;18(1):15-24.

15. Locker GY, Hamilton S, Harris J, et al. ASCO 2006 update of recommendations for the use of tumor markers in gastrointestinal cancer. *J Clin Oncol.* 2006;24(33):5317-5327.

16. Winawer SJ, Stewart ET, Zauber AG, et al. A comparison of colonoscopy and double-contrast barium enema for surveillance after polypectomy. National Polyp Study Work Group. *N Engl J Med.* 2000;342(24): 1766-1772.

17. Pox CP, Schmiegel W. Role of CT colonography in colorectal cancer screening: risks and benefits. *Gut.* 2010;59(5):692-700.

18. Weston BR, Iyer RB, Qiao W, et al. Ability of integrated positron emission and computed tomography to detect significant colonic pathology. *Cancer.* 2010;116(6):1454-1461.

19. Chang JM, Lee HJ, Goo JM, et al. False positive and false negative FDG-PET scans in various thoracic diseases. *Korean J Radiol.* 2006;7(1):57-69.

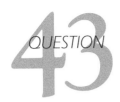

A 78-Year-Old Man With Metastatic Colon Cancer Had a Colonic Stent Placed 16 Months Ago. He Has Developed Recurrent Obstruction at the Site of the Tumor. How Should This Patient Be Evaluated and Managed?

Waqar A. Qureshi, MD and Yasser H. Shaib, MD, MPH, FASGE

This patient had a colonic stent placed for palliation of metastatic colon cancer 16 months ago. He appears to have done very well but now presents with obstruction at the site to the initial tumor. Self-expanding metal stents (SEMS) are placed in the colon for 2 main indications:

1. Palliation in cases of advanced (metastatic) or inoperable colon cancer presenting with bowel obstruction. This group may also include patients with other comorbidities who cannot undergo surgery.

2. As a bridge to elective surgery in patients who present with malignant colon obstruction but are too sick to go directly to surgery. This group has an unacceptably high mortality from emergency surgery when they present with acute obstruction and without formal bowel cleansing.

In the United States, all available colonic stents are uncovered metal mesh devices, some of which are deployed under fluoroscopy alone via large-bore catheters, and others are through-the-scope (TTS) devices deployed under endoscopic and fluoroscopic guidance (Figures 43-1 and 43-2).

Figure 43-1. Fluoroscopic view of a colonic stent immediately following deployment. Note the waist in the middle of the stent, denoting the site of the malignant stenosis.

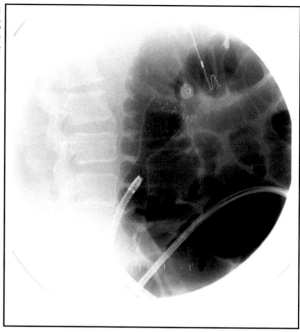

Figure 43-2. Endoscopic image of a colonic stent following deployment.

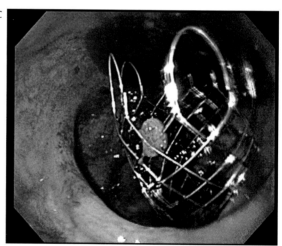

Colonic metal stents have high technical and clinical success rates.[1] Technical success refers to satisfactory placement of the stent at the correct location. Clinical success refers to an improvement in obstructive symptoms, etc. In a study by Small and colleagues, these rates were 96% and 99% in the palliative group and 95% and 98% in the preoperative group, respectively.[2] In this study, complications rates were as follows; perforation (9%), occlusion (9%), migration (5%), and erosion/ulceration (2%), although some authors report lower complication rates.

Most patients with malignant bowel obstruction have left-sided disease, likely due to the frequency of lesions at this location combined with higher stool viscosity in the distal colon. Tumors in the right colon present with obstruction less frequently, as stool has a

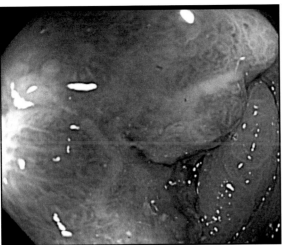

Figure 43-3. Endoscopic image of tumor overgrowth at the distal end of a previously placed colonic stent causing complete large bowel obstruction. No portion of the stent is visible endoscopically. (Reprinted with permission of Douglas G. Adler, MD.)

higher water content in the proximal colon. Although there are fewer data for the use of colon stents in the proximal colon, SEMS seem to be safe and effective at locations proximal to the splenic flexure as well.

In the case being discussed, one or more of the following scenarios is likely to have occurred:

- The tumor has grown through the stent wall interstices and blocked the lumen (tumor ingrowth).
- The tumor has grown over the proximal and/or distal ends of the stent (tumor overgrowth). Figure 43-3 is an endoscopic photograph of this scenario.
- The stent is impacted with stool.
- The stent has migrated more distally, letting more proximal tumor close off the lumen.
- The stent has grown into or perforated through the wall of the colon but is not open to the peritoneum.

Initial management should include hydration and correction of any electrolyte abnormalities. Plain abdominal X-rays should be obtained to rule out free air and record the cecal diameter (a cecum 10 to 12 cm in diameter or larger may be a prelude to perforation). We would obtain a CAT scan to confirm the position of the stent relative to the tumor, evaluate for tumor ingrowth and/or overgrowth, and look for any sign of perforation. We would then perform a colonoscopy with fluoroscopic guidance following laxatives or tap water enemas, because a formal bowel preparation cannot be performed in this patient. One can then see directly if the stent has migrated or is blocked from tumor ingrowth. If the scope cannot traverse the lumen of the stent, as we suspect is likely in this patient, one can inject radio-opaque dye through a catheter to outline the narrowed lumen, give an estimate of the length of the affected lumen, and then pass a guide wire through the stricture to ensure access to the proximal colon. Once guide wire access to the proximal colon has been obtained, the fastest and most effective therapy would be to place a new stent through the existing stent. This would re-canalize the lumen and allow rapid bowel decompression. Balloon dilation of a malignant colonic stricture should in most cases be avoided as it can increase the risk of perforation. If there is extensive tumor ingrowth, laser treatments can be used to ablate tumor to re-canalize the lumen enough to allow the placement of a second SEMS through the first one.

In this patient, if it turns out that the stent has migrated and can be easily and safely removed, we would remove it before attempting to place a new stent across the obstruction. Stent removal can be performed using a rat-tooth forceps or a snare. Sometimes, a partially migrated stent cannot be removed safely due to tumor ingrowth, in which case a much safer option is to simply place a second stent without even attempting to remove the first stent.

In this patient, one would likely see a rapid improvement in his clinical status following placement of a SEMS, most likely through the lumen of the first stent. Patients should be advised to follow a low-residue diet and to take laxatives, stool softeners, or mineral oil supplements to avoid stool impaction after SEMS placement.

If there is any sign of perforation during the pre-endoscopy evaluation of this patient, he should proceed directly to surgery. Similarly, if endoscopy reveals a stent that is completely overgrown with tumor and guide wire access to the proximal colon cannot be obtained, then surgical options are more likely to be successful and should be considered. In addition to effectively managing acute colonic obstruction from malignancy, SEMS placement allows for preoperative (bridge to surgery) and palliative treatment of large bowel obstruction in advanced malignancy.[3] It enables improved quality of life without the need for surgery for palliation.[4]

References

1. Repici A, Adler DG, Gibbs CM, Malesci A, Preatoni P, Baron TH. Stenting of the proximal colon in patients with malignant large bowel obstruction: techniques and outcomes. *Gastrointest Endosc.* 2007;66(5):940-944.
2. Small AJ, Coelho-Prabhu N, Baron TH. Endoscopic placement of self-expandable metal stents for malignant colonic obstruction: long-term outcomes and complication factors. *Gastrointest Endosc.* 2010;71(3):560-572.
3. Alcantara M, Serra X, Bombardó J, et al. Colorectal stenting as an effective therapy for preoperative and palliative treatment of large bowel obstruction: 9 years' experience. *Tech Coloproctol.* 2007;11(4):316-322.
4. Nagula S, Ishill N, Nash C, et al. Quality of life and symptom control after stent placement or surgical palliation of malignant colorectal obstruction. *J Am Coll Surg.* 2010;210(1):45-53.

SECTION VII

RECTUM AND ANUS

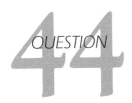

A 55-Year-Old Man Presents With Rectal Bleeding. A Digital Rectal Exam Reveals a Firm 1-cm Perianal Lesion. Biopsy of This Lesion is Consistent With Squamous Cell Carcinoma. How Do You Manage This Patient?

Selvi Thirumurthi, MD, MS

The most common type of anal cancer arises from the squamous epithelium of the distal anal canal. Cancers originating from the proximal anal canal are less common and arise from columnar epithelium. The treatment of these anal adenocarcinomas is very similar to rectal adenocarcinomas. Our patient's biopsy reveals squamous cell carcinoma of the anal canal, and we will focus on this clinical entity.

The most common presenting symptom of anal cancer is anal bleeding followed by the sensation of fullness or a mass. Up to 20% of patients with anal cancer may be asymptomatic. Risk factors for anal cancer include infection with human papilloma virus (HPV) or HIV, a history of sexually transmitted diseases, and history of receptive anal intercourse. Anal cancer can also develop in patients following solid-organ transplant on immunosuppressive medication.[1]

With regard to the natural history of the disease, anal cancer can extend in a bidirectional manner from the anal margin or anal canal into the rectum or to the perianal skin

Figure 44-1. Endoscopic image of an ulcerated anal cancer extending proximally into the distal rectum, viewed from the anal verge with a colonoscope. (Reprinted with permission of Douglas G. Adler, MD.)

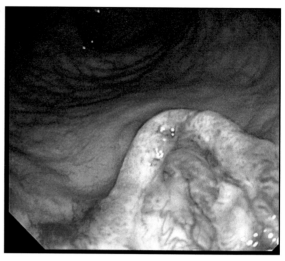

(Figure 44-1). Inguinal and internal iliac lymph nodes that drain the distal and proximal anal canal, respectively, can become involved with metastatic disease. These can be detected on cross-sectional imaging (CT or MRI) or transrectal endoscopic ultrasound (EUS). Distant metastatic disease is uncommon in anal cancer but can include perirectal lymph nodes or hepatic metastases, which can be extensive.

Before we can discuss the treatment options with this patient, we must first determine the stage of his disease. A history and physical exam have been performed with biopsy of the anal lesion. Additional testing includes a proctoscopy, fine-needle aspiration of any enlarged lymph nodes, cross-sectional imaging of the abdomen and pelvis, basic blood work, and an HIV test if indicated by the patient's history. Colonoscopy may be indicated if other symptoms are present or as preoperative clearance to evaluate for internal extension and to rule out any synchronous colonic disease.[2]

The mainstay of anal cancer treatment has historically been abdomino-perineal resection (APR), which results in loss of the anal sphincter and permanent end colostomy. This surgery may be complicated by sexual dysfunction. These outcomes may not be acceptable to our relatively young patient. Fortunately, he has other options. Combination chemotherapy and radiation were previously used as a neoadjuvant treatment modality prior to APR, but the positive outcomes seen in patients receiving this treatment have made these treatments the first-line therapy for most anal cancers. APR is now only indicated in a few clinical situations including the treatment of radiation-induced complications that are discussed below. APR can also be used as salvage therapy when chemotherapy and radiation have failed.[2]

The recommended therapy of anal squamous cell carcinoma, as with any cancer, can change over time based on the best evidence that is available. The primary treatment of anal squamous cell carcinoma currently depends upon whether the lesion is located at the anal margin or in the anal canal according to the 2010 National Comprehensive Cancer Network (NCCN) Clinical Practice Guidelines. Squamous cell carcinomas of the anal canal without metastatic disease are treated with combination chemotherapy (5-fluorouracil and mitomycin) and radiation. Metastatic anal canal cancers are treated with a cisplatin-based chemotherapy regimen alone. Anal margin cancers that are small (less than 2 cm) are treated with wide local excision. If the margins are inadequate, re-excision versus chemotherapy and radiation are options. For tumors larger than 2 cm or those with regional lymph node involvement, 5-fluorouracil and mitomycin with radiation therapy is recommended. Metastatic anal margin cancers are treated with cisplatin-based chemotherapy without radiation.[3]

Combination chemotherapy and radiation offers several advantages. This is a non-invasive treatment modality and saves our patient the morbidity and mortality associated with an APR. In addition, good patient outcomes have been achieved with local control of disease and colostomy-free survival. Local disease recurrence with combination therapy is low, and survival rates up to 90% have been reported. Short-term complications of combination therapy have been reported. These include perineal skin desquamation, nausea, vomiting, diarrhea, cystitis, and vaginitis. Potential long-term complications can occur, including perineal fibrosis and the development of telangiectasias of the rectum (radiation proctitis), bladder, or vagina, which can manifest as bleeding from these organs and which can be difficult to treat. Fecal incontinence as a complication from chemotherapy and radiation therapy occurs in up to 10% of patients, and its development usually warrants treatment via APR.[2]

Conclusion

Anal cancer presents as loco-regional disease in the majority of cases. Combination chemotherapy and radiation therapy has replaced APR as the primary treatment modality, although some patients will still require surgical interventions. Chemotherapy combined with radiation offers a less-invasive, sphincter-sparing approach with good survival and low local recurrence rates. Treatment of patients with anal cancer requires a multidisciplinary approach with the combined efforts of gastroenterologists, surgeons, and medical and radiation oncologists. Our patient can be counseled about the positive outcomes in anal squamous cell carcinoma with currently available therapy in terms of non-invasive treatment modalities (chemotherapy and radiation), avoiding surgery, and excellent survival rates (up to 90%).

References

1. Van Kemseke C. Sexually transmitted diseases and anorectum. *Acta Gastroenterol Belg.* 2009;72(4):413-419.
2. Malik U, Mohiuddin M. Anal cancer. In: Abeloff MD, Armitage JO, eds. Abeloff's clinical oncology. Philadelphia, PA: Churchill Livingstone Elsevier Incorporated; 2008:1557-1567.
3. National Comprehensive Cancer Network. NCCN clinical practice guidelines in oncology. http://www.nccn.org/professionals/physician_gls/f_guidelines.asp. Accessed May 9, 2010.

Why Are Rectal Cancers so Different From Colon Cancers With Regard to Medical and Surgical Management?

Kimberly Jones, MD

The major differences between colon and rectal cancer with regard to treatment are mainly due to the difference in location. Rectal cancers are defined as tumors occurring in the distal 12 cm of the bowel or below the peritoneal reflection intraoperatively (Figure 45-1). The transition point from the sigmoid colon to the rectum is marked by the fusion of the tenia of the sigmoid colon to form the circumferential longitudinal muscle of the rectum. The rectum is also divided into thirds when discussing surgical planning into upper rectal cancer, mid rectal cancers, and distal rectal cancers. Surgery has been the mainstay of therapy for both localized and locally advanced rectal cancer, although surgery alone is curative in only a minority of cases, warranting other therapy. Resection of rectal cancer can be technically challenging due the relative inaccessibility of structures within the pelvis, as well as the desire to preserve anal sphincter function whenever possible while achieving appropriate margins.

In colon cancer, surgeons remove a large portion of bowel and adjacent lymph nodes and can achieve good margins and restore intestinal continuity in the majority of patients. Adequate surgical margins are much more difficult to achieve in rectal cancer, and much higher local recurrence rates and poorer survivals were noted in rectal cancer patients compared to colon cancer. This led to many changes in treatment, including surgery and the use of preoperative (neoadjuvant) radiation and chemotherapy in the majority of patients.

Figure 45-1. Endoscopic image of a large, ulcerating, circumferential rectal cancer 9 cm from the anal verge. The lesion is very likely to be locally advanced on formal staging. (Reprinted with permission of Douglas G. Adler, MD.)

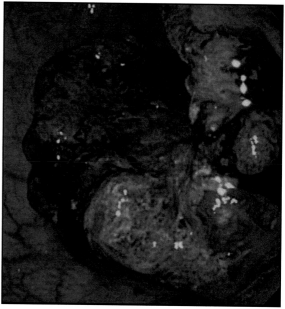

Surgical Options for Rectal Cancer

Prior to 1997, conventional surgical techniques, either abdominoperineal resection (APR) or low anterior resection (LAR), had unacceptable local recurrence rates. Recurrence was likely due to minute foci of adenocarcinoma in the mesorectum several centimeters distal to the apparent lower edge of a rectal cancer.[1] These findings gave rise to the procedure known as total mesorectal excision (TME). This procedure involves a dissection, under direct vision, between the parietal and visceral planes of the pelvic fascia. TME allows for complete resection of an intact rectum along with its surrounding mesorectum, enveloped within the visceral pelvic fascia with a well-defined circumferential margin (CRM). As a result of TME, 5-year survival figures have improved from 45% to 50% to 75%, and local recurrence rates have declined from 30% to 5% to 8%.[2]

Local Recurrence Following Surgery

Despite the improvement in surgical techniques, local recurrence is still a problem when rectal cancer is compared to colon cancer, where local recurrence is relatively rare. Local recurrence in the pelvis is associated with significant pain due to pelvic sidewall or sacral invasion, as well as obstructive symptoms, and may or may not be amendable to repeat resection. Even when potentially resectable, recurrent rectal cancer has a poor prognosis.

Medical Oncology Options for Rectal Cancer Before and After Surgery

Given the data that both adjuvant and neoadjuvant (delivered before surgery) chemotherapy and radiation therapy have been shown to reduce local recurrence and improve

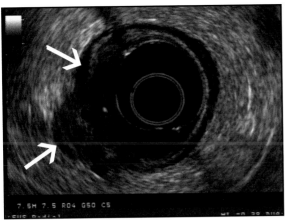

Figure 45-2. A 7.5-MHz radial EUS image of a T3 rectal cancer. Note that the tumor (dark arrow) has breached the muscularis propria (white arrow) and invaded to the level of the adventitia. This patient would receive neoadjuvant therapy prior to surgery. (Reprinted with permission of Douglas G. Adler, MD.)

overall survival, these have now become the standard of care for all locally advanced rectal cancer. The use of preoperative endoscopic ultrasound staging (EUS) is critical in determining which patients have locally advanced disease and are most likely to benefit from neoadjuvant therapy. Pelvic magentic resonance imaging (MRI) is also used to determine local stage and surgical planning.

Tumors appropriate for surgery alone include superficially invasive, low-grade, and small tumor stage 1 lesions. The use of neoadjuvant chemoradiotherapy for T2 lesions remains a topic of controversy. The 5-year overall survival for patients with T1 (mucosal) lesions treated with surgery alone is nearly 100% but drops to 82% in T2 lesions (tumor invades but does not breach the muscularis propria).[3] Furthermore, the risk of nodal metastasis is closely related to T stage, with T1 lesions having an incidence of lymph node metastasis of 12.7%, compared to 19% in T2 tumors.[4]

Identifiable high-risk factors for recurrence of early stage cancers (T1-T2) include poorly differentiated tumors, nonexophytic (ulcerated or flat-raised) tumors, and the presence of lymphvascular invasion.[5] Patients with T3 tumors (that breach the muscularis propria) or who have any evidence of nodal involvement on EUS are recommended to undergo neoadjuvant chemoradiotherapy prior to surgery (Figure 45-2). Patients with T4 tumors may not be amenable to surgery. Besides EUS, staging for both colon cancer and rectal cancer is otherwise the same and should include a computed tomography (CT) scan of the chest, abdomen, and pelvis as well as serum carcinoembryonic antigen (CEA) level. A chest X-ray is not a substitute for a chest CT as both colon and rectal cancers can spread to the lungs and a chest X-ray may miss smaller lesions.

One of the controversial issues in early-stage rectal cancer has been the issue of preoperative versus postoperative chemotherapy or radiotherapy. The main disadvantage of preoperative therapy (neoadjuvant) is primarily the risk of overtreating some patients due to staging inaccuracies and the lack of adequate histopathology. The main disadvantages of postoperative (adjuvant) therapy are related to poor patient tolerance and/or refusal of treatment, as well as delays in initiating postoperative therapy. In our current practice, if a patient has a borderline tumor, a frank discussion of these potential risks and benefits with neoadjuvant therapy is critical to informed decision-making. Patients opting to undergo neoadjuvant therapy are often willing to accept the possibility of overtreatment.

If a patient selects surgery alone and the final pathological staging is higher than had been previously determined, adjuvant chemoradiotherapy is still a reasonable option and would be recommended.

Another area of discussion includes the use of neoadjuvant therapy in an effort to potentially achieve sphincter preservation in patients with distal rectal cancer (lesions that arise less than 5 cm from the anal verge). Data support the idea that neoadjuvant therapy may help preserve sphincter function, so neoadjuvant therapy can be offered to patients with distal rectal tumors or any tumor that would likely require an APR in an attempt for sphincter preservation.

Despite the complexity of the topic, neoadjuvant chemoradiation is currently the favored approach for the treatment of stage II and III rectal cancers and for palliation of local symptoms in metastatic (stage IV) rectal cancer. Neoadjuvant chemotherapy and radiation is given using external beam radiation therapy with either continuous 5-fluorouracil (5-FU) or an oral analog capecitabine (Xeloda) as a radiation sensitizer (which is believed to be at least equivalent to 5-FU and does not require a central line to infuse).

The ability to have a pretreatment clinical stage as well as a final pathological stage is also unique to rectal cancer and provides an excellent marker of therapeutic response and/or treatment sensitivity. Patients who do have complete pathological response have a better prognosis overall. This prognostic information is not available for colon cancer as final T stage and N stage are not known until after surgery. There is no treatment prior to surgery with chemotherapy or radiation so treatment response cannot be evaluated as it is in rectal cancer.

The recommended therapy after resection for rectal cancer versus colon cancer is also different. For some stage II and all stage III colon cancers, we recommend 6 months of postoperative (adjuvant) systemic chemotherapy, ideally with FOLFOX (a regimen containing 5-FU and oxaliplatin). For rectal cancers, the prior standard adjuvant therapy has included an additional 4 to 6 months of chemotherapy with just 5-FU alone. I, as well as others, feel comfortable offering the more intensive therapy (FOLFOX versus 5-FU alone) we use for colon cancer in my patients with high-risk or stage III rectal cancers and discuss the rationale with them. The number of months of treatment remains to be determined and could be less than 6 months, considering these patients often also receive neoadjuvant treatment (chemotherapy given before surgery with radiation), whereas colon cancer patients do not.

Now that therapy for rectal cancer has been modified to account for anatomical differences, we would expect to see the overall survival for colon and rectal cancers to be similar when compared stage by stage. The key differences are the use of EUS for preoperative treatment planning, detailed pelvic resection using TME, and the incorporation of radiotherapy, which are unique to rectal cancer. Patients with rectal cancer may warrant referral to a large cancer center. The chemotherapeutic regimens should be tailored to the individual case. The ability to see the effect of neoadjuvant chemoradiotherapy on rectal cancer may help with the planning of postoperative chemotherapy.

References

1. Scott N, Jackson P, al-Jaberi T, Dixon MF, Quirke P, Finan PJ. Total mesorectal excision and local recurrence: a study of tumour spread in the mesorectum distal to rectal cancer. *Br J Surg.* 1995;82(8):1031-1033.
2. Enker WE. Total mesorectal excision—the new golden standard of surgery for rectal cancer. *Ann Med.* 1997;29(2):127-133.

3. Serra-Aracil X, Vallverdú H, Bombardó-Junca J, Pericay-Pijaume C, Urgellés-Bosch J, Navarro-Soto S. Long-term follow-up of local rectal cancer surgery by transanal endoscopic microsurgery. *World J Surg.* 2008;32(6):1162-1167.

4. Rasheed S, Bowley DM, Aziz O, et al. Can depth of tumour invasion predict lymph node positivity in patients undergoing resection for early rectal cancer? A comparative study between T1 and T2 cancers. *Colorectal Dis.* 2008;10(3):231-238.

5. Chambers WM, Khan U, Gagliano A, Smith RD, Sheffield J, Nicholls RJ. Tumour morphology as a predictor of outcome after local excision of rectal cancer. *Br J Surg.* 2004;91(4):457-459.

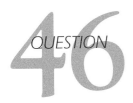
What Is the Role of Endorectal Ultrasound in Patients With Rectal Cancer? Do All Patients With Rectal Cancer Need to Have an Endorectal Ultrasound?

Leyla J. Ghazi, MD and David A. Schwartz, MD

Transrectal endosonography (EUS) has emerged as a critical imaging modality for pre-treatment staging of rectal cancer. The role of EUS has further expanded with the introduction of EUS-guided fine-needle aspiration (FNA) of intramural and extramural lesions, as well as extra-luminal abnormalities. EUS staging of rectal cancers is performed in an effort to identify the subgroup of patients who may benefit from preoperative chemoradiotherapy prior to operative intervention. The advantage of preoperative treatment is to downsize the tumor in an attempt to facilitate sphincter preservation, reduce or eliminate local adenopathy, decrease local recurrence, and improve survival. Staging using the standardized tumor, lymph nodes, and metastases (ie, TNM) classification system is usually performed to guide treatment decisions and prognosis. The primary variable that affects outcomes in rectal cancer is the loco-regional pathologic staging of the tumor, including the depth of tumor invasion (T-stage) and the presence of metastatic lymph nodes (N-stage).

The relationship between survival and depth of tumor invasion has been well-established. The 5-year survival rates of early cancers (T0) are as high as 95%, whereas advanced cancers (T2-3) have survival rates as low as 25% to 60%. EUS is a safe and accurate diagnostic method that allows assessment of tumor invasion into the rectal wall and its associated lymph node status.[1] At our institution, we use a radial echoendoscope, which can be advanced under direct visualization above the level of the lesion to a point where the

---

Table 46-1

The Ultrasonographic Staging Corresponding to Tumor, Lymph Nodes, and Metastases Classification

Stage	T Groups	Wall Layer
Stage 0	T0 (Tis)	Carcinoma in situ; confined to mucosa or mm[1]
Stage I or IIIA*	T1	Invades submucosa; does not invade mp[2]
Stage I, IIIA*, IIIB*	T2	Invades mp[2]
Stage IIA or IIIB*	T3	Beyond mp[2]; infiltrating perirectal fat
Stage IIB, IIC, or IIIB*	T4	Infiltrates surrounding organs

Stage IIIC and IV are reserved for N2M0 and NXM1 disease, respectively.
[1]Muscularis mucosa.
[2]Muscularis propria.
*Depending upon nodal status.

---

iliac vessels and lymph nodes can be assessed. A dedicated pass of the echoendoscope should be reserved for lymph node inspection. In our experience, the presence of identifiable lymph nodes on EUS in the perirectal region is suggestive of malignant invasion. In general, because of the high probability for metastatic involvement when lymph nodes are visualized, we perform FNA of lymph nodes only in the subgroup of patients for whom the results can impact preoperative management, such as those with early T-stage disease (ie, T1, 2). The risk of lymph node metastases increases from 10% to 79% with increasing tumor T-stage (T1-4). Malignant nodes are more likely to be round, well-demarcated, hypoechoic, and greater than 1 cm in size. Not all malignant nodes have this appearance, and any suspicious-appearing node can be sampled via EUS-guided FNA.[2]

When looking at the tumor itself, the endosonographer should perform a meticulous examination of the contour and thickness of the rectal wall, followed by an assessment of the depth of tumor penetration. Staging accuracy can sometimes be improved by instilling water into the rectal lumen. This allows for acoustic coupling without direct compression of the tumor by the ultrasound probe, which can sometimes lead to over-staging. The bowel wall is identified as five distinct alternating hyper- and hypoechoic layers corresponding to the histologic layers (mucosa, muscularis mucosa, submucosa, muscularis propria, and serosa). Carcinomas are typically hypoechoic, and the degree to which they disrupt and penetrate the rectal wall layers suggests local or advanced stage disease (Table 46-1).

Based upon the TNM classification system, T0 tumors are confined to the mucosa. These can also be categorized as carcinoma in situ and are not felt to have metastatic potential. T1 tumors invade the submucosa; endosonographically, a focal hypoechoic mass is typically seen in contact with the lamina propria or submucosa without evidence of invasion into the muscularis propria (Figure 46-1). T2 tumors invade into, but do not go through, the muscularis propria (Figure 46-2). In these patients, the muscularis propria

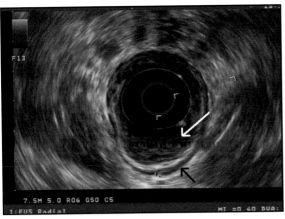

Figure 46-1. EUS image of a T1 rectal cancer. Note that the mass (white arrow) does not breach or distort the muscularis propria (black arrow). (Reprinted with permission of Douglas G. Adler, MD.)

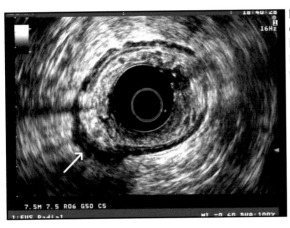

Figure 46-2. EUS image of a T2 rectal cancer. Note the thickening and irregularity of the muscularis propria deep to the mass (arrow). (Reprinted with permission of Douglas G. Adler, MD.)

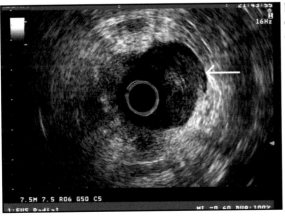

Figure 46-3. EUS image of a T3 rectal cancer. The muscularis propria has been obliterated by the mass (arrow), and this wall layer is no longer visible. (Reprinted with permission of Douglas G. Adler, MD.)

may appear thickened or irregular, suggesting invasion. T3 tumors invade through the muscularis propria and infiltrate the perirectal fat (Figure 46-3). T4 tumors invade surrounding organs and structures (Figure 46-4). Last, examination of the anal sphincter can detect loss of continuity of and tumor penetration into the external and internal sphincters. These findings can be valuable in the evaluation of patients with associated fecal incontinence.[1,3]

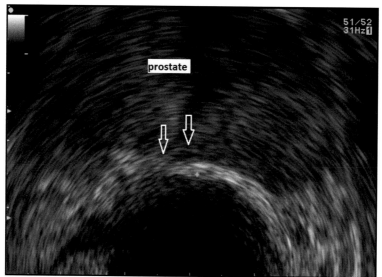

Figure 46-4. EUS image of a T4 cancer seen to be invading the adjacent prostate gland. The arrows point to an area of microinvasion.

Other modalities that have been used for the TNM staging of rectal cancer include magnetic resonance imaging (MRI) and computerized tomography (CT) scan imaging. The T-staging accuracy of EUS has surpassed that of both MRI and CT scan; however, in general, nodal identification has been suboptimal across all imaging modalities. Most studies looking at EUS FNA use have shown significantly improved accuracy. A recent meta-analysis of all EUS studies from 1998 to 2008 showed a 88% to 95% accuracy, with improved sensitivity and specificity in the early (T1) and advanced stage cancers (T3 and T4). The sensitivity and specificity of EUS in diagnosing nodal involvement is around 75%, similar to that seen in MRI imaging. In general, overstaging (especially with T2 lesions) is more frequent than understaging.[4]

The expertise of the operator also plays a role in accuracy. Studies suggest a learning curve of up to 50 cases for the ability to correctly assess tumor depth and more than 75 cases for accurate node status assessments. Interpretation of sonography is often more difficult after manipulation of the tumor by attempts at endoscopic excision or following chemoradiation therapy. Inflammation, edema, and bleeding can cause obliteration of the sonographic layers and make accurate staging assessment difficult. A common dilemma is the staging of a cancer that has been endoscopically biopsied via techniques that use electrocautery, such as "hot" snares or biopsy forceps. The electrocautery induces significant artifact that can frequently result in overstaging.

All patients with rectal cancer may not be able to undergo an endosonographic evaluation. A tight rectal stricture that precludes insertion of the echoendoscope beyond the tumor may prevent adequate examination of the rectal wall. Other potential contraindications to endosonography may include the presence of perforation or microperforations. Furthermore, endosonographic staging may not be required for patients with early-stage disease (T0), documented tumors on a stalk after complete resection, and advanced-stage disease (stage 4) for whom an operative approach is not indicated.

EUS has become the diagnostic tool of choice for the pre-treatment staging of rectal cancer. The accuracy of this modality is dependent on multiple factors including operator expertise, peritumoral inflammation, and edema, and is complicated by the potential for overstaging. However, the precision of T-staging via EUS is superior compared to other available imaging modalities with similar N-staging accuracy.

References

1. Schaffzin DM, Wong WD. Endorectal ultrasound in the preoperative evaluation of rectal cancer. *Clin Colorectal Cancer.* 2004;4(2):124-132.
2. Harewood GC, Wiersema MJ, Nelson H, et al. A prospective, blinded assessment of the impact of preoperative staging on the management of rectal cancer. *Gastroenterology.* 2002;123(1):24-32.
3. Kav T, Bayraktar Y. How useful is rectal endosonography in the staging of rectal cancer? *World J Gastroenterol.* 2010;16(6):691-697.
4 Puli SR, Reddy JBK, Bechtold ML, Choudhary A, Antillon MR, Brugge WR. How good is endoscopic ultrasound in differentiating various T stages of rectal cancer? Meta-analysis and systematic review. *Ann Surg Oncol.* 2009;16(2):254-265.

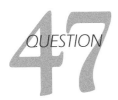
WHICH PATIENTS WITH RECTAL CANCER SHOULD UNDERGO NEOADJUVANT THERAPY AND WHICH PATIENTS CAN PROCEED DIRECTLY TO SURGERY?

Ryan C. Van Woerkom, MD
and Douglas G. Adler, MD, FACG, AGAF, FASGE

Colorectal cancer (CRC) is the third leading cause of death in the United States of men and women. The rectum lies between the anogenital ring and extends into the rectosigmoid junction. Adenocarcinoma developing at the distal 12 to 15 cm of the colon is typically depicted as rectal cancer. As defined, 40,870 Americans will develop rectal cancer (RC) according to the American Cancer Society's newest estimated incidence in 2009 for the United States.[1,2] Advancing age, a family history of CRC or polyps, a personal history of inflammatory bowel disease, pelvic radiation therapy, or inherited genetic mutations such as hereditary nonpolyposis CR, familial adenomatous polyposis, Turcot's, Gardner's, Peutz-Jeghers, Muir-Torre, juvenile polyposis syndromes, and traditional modifiable risk factors all increase the risk of RC.[3]

Imaging

Magnetic resonance imaging (MRI), endoscopic ultrasound (EUS), and computed tomography (CT) are used in the evaluation of RCs, but each has its own limitations. MRI excludes patients with specific metal prostheses, and EUS can't be used if the rectal lesion causes profound stenosis; both of these studies are not available at all institutions. Comparison of the three imaging modalities consistently demonstrates that CT is not as accurate as diagnosing tumor invasion through the wall of the rectum. Modern imaging techniques have led to improvements in specific-stage treatments in rectal cancer.

Table 47-1

Management of Rectal Cancer Against Stratified Rectal Cancer Stages

Cancer Stage/ Management Option	TME alone	Neoadjuvant radiochemotherapy	Adjuvant therapy
Tis, T0, T1, T2, N0	Viable option	No, except possibly in T2 lesions	Possible pending operative findings
High-risk T2, T3, T4, N1, distal tumor	Surgery followed only after neoadjuvant therapy	Yes, especially in cases of sphincter sparing	Chemotherapy alone
M1	For palliative care	For palliative care	Not available

Neoadjuvant Therapy Versus Surgery Alone

Surgery has historically been the chief therapeutic option for rectal cancer but is only curative in a minority of cases.[4] Rectal cancer resection can be technically challenging due to tumor location deep in the pelvis and desire to preserve anal sphincter function. Improvements in surgical technique, specifically total mesorectal excision (TME), have reduced recurrence rates, improved survival rates, and reduced the rates of impotence and bladder dysfunction.[5] TME is now the standard of care in clinical practice.

The following types of rectal cancer are suited for surgery alone: local low-grade small tumors (tumor stage [T] Tis, T0, T1, T2, all being N0) that are superficially invasive or American Joint Committee on Cancer (AJCC) stage I lesions. T2 lesions still remain a controversial topic because the 5-year overall survival rate for T1 is almost 100% while T2 drifts down to 82%, often due to involved local nodes (Table 47-1).[6] Additionally, nodal metastasis relates closely to T stage. Currently identified risk factors for recurrence of early-stage cancers (T1-T2) include poorly differentiated tumors, nonexophytic (flat-raised or ulcerated) tumors, and the presence of lymphovascular invasion by the tumor.

With the improvement of surgical treatment, neoadjuvant therapy in the treatment of rectal cancer or chemo-radiotherapy is generally selected for those patients who have locally advanced lesions. Tumor response to neoadjuvant therapy may help determine recommendations for postoperative adjuvant therapy. Less irradiation-induced bowel injury, fewer toxic side effects, and better compliance are seen with neoadjuvant chemotherapy as compared with postoperative (adjuvant) chemo-radiotherapy.

Available Data Regarding Neoadjuvant Therapy for Rectal Cancer

The Erlangen Registry of Colorectal Carcinoma (ERCRC) demonstrated that patients with T3 tumors could be further divided into risk according to the maximal tumor invasion beyond the outer border of the muscularis propria—a histologic measurement: Tumors with less than 5 mm of invasion and those with greater than 5 mm of invasion were in the low- and high-risk categories, respectively. Local recurrence rates were higher, and cancer-related 5-year mortality rates were lower in the higher-risk category, but once these categories were adjusted for lymph node involvement, the 5-year survival rates were similar.[7]

The main disadvantage of preoperative (neoadjuvant) therapy is the risk of overtreating someone primarily due to the staging inaccuracies and lack of adequate histopathology. Major disadvantages of postoperative (adjuvant) therapy include poor patient compliance and/or tolerance as well as delays in initiating adjuvant chemo-radiotherapy. The German Rectal Trial including 799 rectal cancer patients randomized to receive either neoadjuvant or adjuvant 5-fluorouracil (5-FU)-based chemoradiotherapy was unable to meet its primary endpoint of increased survival in neoadjuvant therapy, although secondary endpoint data including rates of disease-free survival, local and distant recurrence, acute and long-term toxic effects, sphincter preservation, and postoperative complications were promising.

Nevertheless, other similar trials have replicated positive benefits of neoadjuvant therapy. The Swedish Rectal Cancer Trial randomized 1168 patients with resectable rectal cancer to high-dose preoperative radio-chemotherapy or surgery alone. This study demonstrated local control of tumor recurrence and improved survival across all subgroups. The Dutch Colorectal Cancer Group more clearly defined the role of preoperative radiotherapy. It included 1784 patients randomized to either neoadjuvant radiotherapy followed by TME or TME alone. This study demonstrated a decreased 2-year failure rate with the addition of neoadjuvant radiotherapy on even a short treatment regimen. A second post-TME trial conducted by the Medical Research Council (CR07) randomized 1350 patients with resectable rectal cancer to either a short course of radiotherapy and TME or TME followed by selective adjuvant chemoradiation therapy. In this study, it demonstrated a decrease in local relapse rates and improved disease-free survival at 3 years. Based on the latter two large trials, neoadjuvant radiotherapy was felt to reduce recurrence rates when compared with TME alone.

Using neoadjuvant therapy to potentially achieve sphincter preservation in patients with distal rectal cancer remains another area of controversy. If a cancer arises from less than 5 cm from the anal verge, this is referred to as distal rectal cancer. Some studies have shown, among patients who underwent abdominoperineal resection (APR), up to 44% to 77% of patients could have sphincter function preserved.[8-11] Overall, neoadjuvant chemoradiation therapy is currently favored for managing stage II and III rectal cancers.

A patient's pretreatment clinical stage as obtained by imaging modalities may be different from the post-treatment stage. Repeat imaging may be warranted in some cases, but the gold standard is pathologic staging. "Tumor downstaging" describes patients with evidence of tumor regression, which gives a final pathologic stage that is lower than a patient's pre-existing clinical stage. Some data suggest tumor downstaging is a more accurate predictor of outcome than the pre-existing clinical stage, response to treatment, or combined clinical stage and response to therapy.[12]

Overall, neoadjuvant therapy plays a critical role in patients with locally advanced rectal cancer, and patients should undergo accurate staging and be made aware of all treatment options before initiating any course of therapy.

References

1. Jemal A, Siegel R, Ward E, et al. Cancer statistics, 2009. *CA Cancer J Clin.* 2009;59(4):225-249.
2. Julien LA, Thorson AG. Current neoadjuvant strategies in rectal cancer. *J Surg Oncol.* 2010;101(4):321-326.
3. Moore JC, Jones KA, Adler DG. Preoperative evaluation of rectal cancer: I. Evaluation, diagnosis, and staging. *Community Oncology.* 2009;6(4):161-165.
4. Ricciardi R, Madoff RD, Rothenberger DA, Baxter NN. Population-based analyses of lymph node metastases in colorectal cancer. *Clin Gastroenterol Hepatol.* 2006;4(12):1522-1527.
5. Kockerling F, Reymond MA, Altendorf-Hofmann A, et al. Influence of surgery on metachronous distant metastases and survival in rectal cancer. *J Clin Oncol.* 1998;16(1):324-329.
6. Serra-Aracil X, Vallverdú H, Bombardó-Junca J, Pericay-Pijaume C, Urgellés-Bosch J, Navarro-Soto S. Long-term follow-up of local rectal cancer surgery by transanal endoscopic microsurgery. *World J Surg.* 2008;32(6):1162-1167.
7. Lieberman DA, Prindiville S, Weiss DG, Willett W. VA Cooperative Study Group 380. Risk factors for advanced colonic neoplasia and hyperplastic polyps in asymptomatic individuals. *JAMA.* 2003;290(22):2959-2967.
8. Rouanet P, Saint-Aubert B, Lemanski C, et al. Restorative and nonrestorative surgery for low rectal cancer after high-dose radiation: long-term oncologic and functional results. *Dis Colon Rectum.* 2002;45(3):305-313.
9. Wagman R, Minsky BD, Cohen AM, Guillem JG, Paty PP. Sphincter preservation in rectal cancer with preoperative radiation therapy and coloanal anastomosis: long term follow-up. *Int J Radiat Oncol Biol Phys.* 1998;42(1):51-57.
10. Hyams DM, Mamounas EP, Petrelli N, et al. A clinical trial to evaluate the worth of preoperative multimodality therapy in patients with operable carcinoma of the rectum: a progress report of National Surgical Breast and Bowel Project Protocol R-03. *Dis Colon Rectum.* 1997;40(2):131-139.
11. Valentini V, Coco C, Cellini N, et al. Ten years of preoperative chemoradiation for extraperitoneal T3 rectal cancer: acute toxicity, tumor response, and sphincter preservation in three consecutive studies. *Int J Radiat Oncol Biol Phys.* 2001;51(2):371-383.
12. Quah HM, Chou JF, Gonen M, et al. Pathologic stage is most prognostic of disease free survival in locally advanced rectal cancer patients after preoperative chemoradiation. *Cancer.* 2008;113(1):57-64.

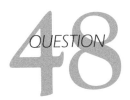

How Should Patients Be Followed After Successful Treatment for Rectal Cancer?

Brad Shepherd, MD; David A. Schwartz, MD; and Paul E. Wise, MD

More than 40,000 people are diagnosed with rectal cancer annually in the United States. Fortunately, survival rates for those with rectal cancer have improved dramatically with new advances in imaging, surgical techniques, and chemotherapeutic regimens. Although 75% of rectal cancer patients present with localized disease that may be amenable to surgical resection, up to 40% of these patients will develop local recurrent or metastatic cancer.[1] There are a number of diagnostic modalities used in postoperative surveillance of rectal cancer with the primary objective of these tests being to detect disease recurrence early in its course. As most recurrence occurs within 2 years of therapy, clinical outcomes may be improved if disease is detected at an early (local) stage. Thus, most accepted protocols for surveillance emphasize aggressive early surveillance with physician visits, imaging, and laboratory analysis. Surveillance recommendations will be impacted somewhat by the initial surgical intervention (eg, transanal excision, radical resection with sphincter preservation, radical resection with permanent colostomy, etc) and use of neoadjuvant or adjuvant therapies (eg, chemoradiation therapy, etc).[2] In this chapter we discuss the basic tenets of rectal cancer surveillance after resection.

Despite the fact that ideal frequency and duration of regular physician follow-up visits after rectal cancer resection has never been formally tested, it is our practice to follow-up with patients every 3 months for the first 2 years after treatment. At that point, routine clinician visits every 6 months for up to 5 years is recommended. The need for further follow-up beyond surveillance endoscopy at this point is left to the discretion of the patient and physician. It is felt that longer follow-up may be required for locally advanced rectal cancer or patients with poor prognostic factors such as lymph node involvement, lymphovascular invasion, poor differentiation, or perineural invasion. Each clinic visit should focus on patient symptoms related to recurrent cancer (eg, hematochezia, weight loss, abdominal pain or changes in bowel habits).

Carcinoembryonic antigen (CEA) is a tumor-associated antigen expressed by most colorectal adenocarcinomas and has value as a tumor marker in those patients with known cancer. Despite the fact that up to 30% of colorectal cancers do not produce CEA, it is still widely used to monitor patients for recurrent disease after curative resection. Although CEA is not used as a screening tool, in those patients with established disease, the CEA level does correlate well with disease burden and offers prognostic value.[3] CEA levels should return to baseline if complete resection is achieved. In patients who are candidates for surgical resection or systemic chemotherapy, those with stage II or III lesions should have postoperative CEA testing done every 3 to 6 months for the first 2 years, then every 6 months for a total of 5 years.[3] Other than routine CEA levels, there is no data to suggest that routine blood tests such as CBC or liver tests are helpful in the post-operative surveillance in these patients.

Endoscopic surveillance after resection for rectal cancer is essential to detect and localize metachronous lesions or anastomotic recurrence at an early stage. Periodic post-treatment surveillance is recommended by the American Society of Clinical Oncology, American Cancer Society, as well as the American Gastroenterological Association. All patients should undergo perioperative colonoscopy to exclude synchronous lesions either preoperatively or within 6 months of resection. At that point, we recommend routine colonoscopic surveillance at 1 year after resection.[4] If this exam is normal, then repeat endoscopy at 3 years and then at 5-year intervals is recommended, assuming no concern for a hereditary colorectal cancer syndrome (eg, familial adenomatous polyposis or hereditary nonpolyposis colorectal cancer) or inflammatory bowel disease exists, which would necessitate more frequent exams. Due to the concern for anastamotic recurrence, proctosigmoidoscopy also has a role in rectal cancer patients. The National Comprehensive Cancer Network (NCCN) guidelines recommend that proctosigmoidoscopy be considered every 6 months for 5 years in rectal cancer patients who underwent low anterior resection (LAR).[4] There is some thought that, in those patients who underwent pelvic radiation and/or after appropriate total mesorectal excision, the use of interval proctosigmoidoscopy is not necessary given their decreased likelihood of local cancer recurrence.

Abdominal imaging with computed tomography (CT) scanning has a role in patients with a high risk for colon or rectal cancer. A survival benefit has been shown in those patients undergoing abdominal imaging at regular intervals when compared to those patients who do not undergo routine imaging.[5] This survival benefit is most pronounced in patients who were able to undergo a curative operation, typically those patients with early stage recurrence. At our institution, we do not routinely obtain abdominal imaging unless CEA levels or clinical circumstances raise suspicion for cancer recurrence. The NCCN does not recommend CT scanning for routine rectal cancer surveillance, just those patients with poor prognostic features as noted previously.[4] ASCO also recommends that patients who are at a high risk of recurrence and who are surgical candidates undergo annual CT scan (ideally of the chest, abdomen, and pelvis) for 3 years after primary therapy.[5] Though there is less evidence for surveillance chest CT in rectal cancer, Chau, et al showed that a larger proportion of resectable recurrences were found on chest imaging compared to abdominal imaging.[3] In addition, pulmonary lesions were as common as liver lesions in rectal cancer patients and were less likely to have elevated CEA levels. Therefore, it is considered appropriate to have high risk patients undergo yearly CT scanning of the chest, abdomen and pelvis yearly for 3 years after resection.

There are few data to support the use of PET scans in routine surveillance of colon and rectal cancer. Thus far, studies on routine PET imaging after rectal cancer treatment have high false-positive and false-negative rates, and the overall survival impact in these patients is questionable.[5] Accordingly, we do not order PET scans unless we have evidence of a rising CEA level and a CT scan that suggests possible (but not definitive) local or distant recurrence or does not suggest obvious recurrent disease. PET scans should be obtained if they are ultimately going to affect the management of the patient (eg, to rule out distant metastasis in the setting of local rectal cancer recurrence).

More recently, there has been an interest in rectal endoscopic ultrasound (EUS) for detection of early local recurrence of rectal cancer.[6] Numerous studies have proven that EUS can be a cost-effective, beneficial means of detecting local cancer recurrence.[1] Morken et al demonstrated that the sensitivity and specificity of EUS in detecting recurrent disease was 87% and 100%, respectively.[7] Additionally, EUS with fine-needle aspiration (FNA) has been shown to identify up to one-third of asymptomatic local recurrences that were missed by digital examination or proctoscopic examination.[7] The major limitation to EUS-guided surveillance is the difficulty in distinguishing postoperative changes and inflammation from recurrent disease, even with use of FNA. There is no consensus as to the frequency of EUS for rectal cancer recurrence surveillance. If EUS is to be used postoperatively, we recommend a post-treatment EUS 3 months after surgery to establish a baseline. This may minimize the chance of misinterpreting postoperative inflammatory changes as recurrent disease because, by this time, most treatment-related changes have stabilized. Recommendations do exist that call for EUS surveillance at 3-month intervals for 2 years followed by 6-month intervals until 3 years post-surgery. While not in widespread use, these recommendations do provide a framework for centers that have the availability to do EUS. The NCCN has not advocated the use of EUS for routine rectal cancer surveillance.[4]

An intensive postoperative surveillance regimen after treatment for rectal cancer, regardless of the initial treatments or surgical intervention, increases the likelihood of surgical resection in the event of recurrent disease. Our summary recommendations are presented in Table 48-1. Despite these recommendations, controversy remains as to the exact timing and nature of this surveillance regimen. Local recurrences generally portend a poor outcome, and it is reasonable to assume that early detection would provide more therapeutic options compared to later recurrence detection, though there are few survival data to support this claim. Undoubtedly, there is a need for large, well-designed clinical trials to better define the most optimal surveillance regimen for this important group of patients.

Table 48-1

Summary Recommendations for Surveillance Following Surgical Treatment for Rectal Cancer

- History and physical exam every 3 to 6 months for 2 years, then every 6 months for 5 years.

- CEA every 3 to 6 months for 2 years, then every 6 months for 5 years for T2 or greater.

- CT chest/abdomen/pelvis annually for 3 years if high risk of recurrence.

- Colonoscopy at 1 year if no preoperative exam
  ○ If advanced adenoma detected, repeat in 1 year
  ○ If no advanced adenoma detected, repeat in 3 years, then every 5 years

- Consider proctoscopy every 6 months x 5 years for post-LAR points.

- PET-CT not recommended for general use but can be considered if CEA rising and clinical suspicion is high.

References

1. Jemal A, Siegel R, Ward E, Hao Y, Xu J, Thun MJ. Cancer statistics, 2009. *CA Cancer J Clin.* 2009;59(4): 225-249.
2. Guillem JG, Paty PB, Cohen AM. Surgical treatment of colorectal cancer. *CA Cancer J Clin.* 1997;47(2): 113-128.
3. Chau I, Allen MJ, Cunningham K, et al. The value of routine serum carcino-embryonic antigen measurement and computed tomography in the surveillance of patients after adjuvant chemotherapy for colorectal cancer. *J Clin Oncol.* 2004;22(8):1420-1429.
4. National Comprehensive Cancer Network. NCCN clinical practice guidelines in oncology 2010: rectal cancer v.3.2011. http://www.nccn.org/professionals/physician_gls/f_guidelines.asp. Accessed April 1, 2010.
5. Desch C, Benson AB III, Somerfield MR, et al. Colorectal cancer surveillance: 2005 update of an American Society of Clinical Oncology Practice Guideline. *J Clin Oncol.* 2005;23(33):8512-8519.
6. de Anda HE, Lee SH, Finne CO, Rothenberger DA, Madoff RD, Garcia-Aguilar J. Endorectal ultrasound in the follow-up of rectal cancer patients treated by local excision or radical surgery. *Dis Colon Rectum.* 2004;47(6):818-824.
7. Morken JJ, Baxter NN, Madoff, RD, Finne CO III. Endorectal ultrasound-directed biopsy: a useful technique to detect local recurrence of rectal cancer. *Int J Colorectal Dis.* 2006;21(3):258-264.

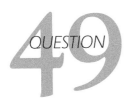

How Low in the Rectum Can a Colonic Stent Be Safely Placed? What Happens if the Stent Is Deployed Too Far Distally?

Vivek Kaul, MD, FACG

Enteral stents are increasingly being used as a non-surgical alternative for the palliation of luminal gastrointestinal neoplasms. During the past decade, endoscopic self-expanding metal stents (SEMS) for obstructing colorectal neoplasms have been widely used for palliation of malignant large bowel obstruction or as a "bridge" to surgery.[1] The development of "through the scope" (TTS) stent delivery systems has facilitated successful stent placement not only in the recto-sigmoid but also in the more proximal colon.[2,3] An important issue to consider in these patients is the feasibility of, and potential problems related to, placement of SEMS low in the rectum, particularly in the region of the ano-rectum. In many instances, the distal extent of an obstructing rectal neoplasm approaches the anal canal and/or abuts the dentate line. In such settings, the distal flare of the stent may rest within 5 cm of the anal verge. This chapter discusses the feasibility of, and potential issues related to, placement of SEMS in such cases.

How Low in the Rectum Can a Metal Stent Be Placed?

In patients with low rectal tumors, the distal flared metal ends of the stent can cause pain, tenesmus, mucosal ulceration, and bleeding, especially when the stent is in contact with the ano-rectum. For these reasons, placement of a SEMS within 5 cm of the anal verge has been traditionally considered a relative contraindication.

Figure 49-1. Endoscopic image of a low lying rectal stent placed in a patient with metastatic ovarian cancer with extrinsic large bowel compression. Note lack of visible tumor due to extrinsic nature of malignancy. The distal end of the stent is within 5 cm of the anal verge. The patient did not develop pain or incontinence following placement. (Reprinted with permission of Douglas G. Adler, MD.)

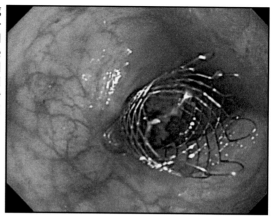

Figure 49-2. Fluoroscopic image of a low lying rectal stent in a patient with metastatic rectal cancer. The distal end of the stent is approximately 4 cm above the anal verge. The patient tolerated the stent well. (Reprinted with permission of Douglas G. Adler, MD.)

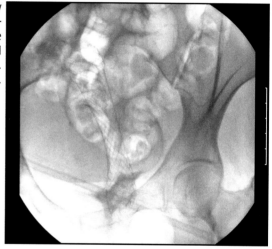

On occasion, especially in women with pelvic/gynecologic cancers, large-mass lesions that extrinsically compress the large bowel can result in very distal large bowel obstructions. In general, these patients are poor operative candidates, and other means of treatment are sought. In carefully selected patients, placement of stents in the distal rectum can be well-tolerated (Figure 49-1).

It is important to have an adequate pre-procedure discussion with any patient with a known rectal obstruction prior to embarking on stent placement. A frank discussion of the risks and benefits of stenting is very helpful. Many patients will accept the risk of some ano-rectal pain or possible incontinence to relieve symptoms of bowel obstruction (which can often be severe and debilitating). In addition, many patients adapt or accommodate to low lying stents over time and learn to adjust their bowel habits to the presence of the prosthesis, further suggesting that, while potentially more problematic, many patients can be well-treated with low-lying colonic stents (Figure 49-2).

Song and colleagues addressed this question in a series of 30 patients with malignant rectal obstruction within 25 mm to 75 mm of the anal verge.[4] The distal ends of the stents were placed within 10 to 30 mm of the anal verge (Group A, n = 16) or within 28 to 50 mm of the anal verge (Group B, n = 14). Ten of 16 patients in Group A had rectal pain/

foreign body sensation, but all were managed with analgesics; comparatively, 1 of 14 patients in Group B had similar symptoms, again, managed with analgesics. Stent migration resulting in severe pain refractory to analgesics required stent removal in a total of 4 patients. The stents used included 3 different types: polyurethane, PTFE, and dual nylon/nitinol. This study demonstrated that although rectal stents can be placed within 5 cm of the anal verge, pain and foreign-body sensation may occur and can generally be managed with analgesics. Stent migration distally toward the ano-rectum will often result in intractable pain and discomfort, requiring stent removal.

A recent report describes placement of the stent too far distally in the anorectum and subsequent management by "trimming" of the distal few centimeters of the nitinol stent using Argon Plasma Coagulation (APC).[5] This was done successfully without any mucosal trauma, and the patient has remained asymptomatic since, but not all stents can be trimmed using this technique. Other authors have described similar management of low rectal stents using APC in a patient with rectal pain.[6]

Conclusion

SEMS placement for malignant colorectal obstruction has high technical success rates and several advantages compared to surgical intervention. Recent data suggest that SEMS can be placed with the distal end very low in the rectum with good clinical outcomes and acceptable risks. If patients with a low lying SEMS experience pain, symptoms are generally manageable with oral analgesics. If the SEMS is deployed too far distally, then options include immediate removal or APC trimming of the distal few centimeters to a custom length. As with any intervention, a detailed discussion with the patient and the multidisciplinary colorectal team regarding all potential aspects of management in a particular situation will usually result in the best outcome.

References

1. Sebastian S, Johnston S, Geoghegan T, Torreggiani W, Buckley M. Pooled analysis of the efficacy and safety of self-expanding metal stenting in malignant colorectal obstruction. *Am J Gastroenterol.* 2004;99(10):2051-2057.
2. Small AJ, Coelho-Prabhu N, Baron TH. Endoscopic placement of self-expandable metal stents for malignant colonic obstruction: long-term outcomes and complication factors. *Gastrointest Endosc.* 2010;71(3):560-572.
3. Repici A, Adler DG, Gibbs CM, Malesci A, Preatoni P, Baron T. Stenting of the proximal colon in patients with malignant large bowel obstruction: techniques and outcomes. *Gastrointest Endosc.* 2007;66(5):940-944.
4. Song HY, Kim J, Kim KR, et al. Malignant rectal obstruction within 5 cm of the anal verge: is there a role for expandable metallic stent placement? *Gastrointest Endosc.* 2008;68(4):713-720.
5. Witte T, Danovitch S, Borum M, Irani S. Endoscopic trimming of a rectal self-expanding metallic stent by use of argon plasma coagulation. *Gastrointest Endosc.* 2007;60(1):210-211.
6. Rao KV, Beri GD, Wang WW. Trimming of a migrated metal stent for malignant colonic stricture using argon plasma coagulation. *World J Gastrointest Endosc.* 2010;2(2):75-76.

FINANCIAL DISCLOSURES

Dr. Douglas G. Adler is a consultant for Boston Scientific, Merit, and Beacon Endoscopy.

Dr. Harshinie C. Amaratunge has no financial or proprietary interest in the materials presented herein.

Dr. Nikhil Banerjee has not disclosed any relevant financial relationships.

Dr. Todd H. Baron receives travel support and is on the speaker's bureau for Cook Endoscopy and Boston Scientific.

Dr. Devina Bhasin has no financial or proprietary interest in the materials presented herein.

Dr. Allene Salcedo Burdette has no financial or proprietary interest in the materials presented herein.

Dr. Clifford S. Cho has no financial or proprietary interest in the materials presented herein.

Dr. David Chu has no financial or proprietary interest in the materials presented herein.

Dr. Peter Darwin has no financial or proprietary interest in the materials presented herein.

Dr. Ananya Das receives an honorarium from the American Society for Gastrointestinal Endoscopy for her role as the Associate Editor of *Gastrointestinal Endoscopy*.

Dr. Christopher J. DiMaio is a consultant for Boston Scientific.

Dr. John Fang has no financial or proprietary interest in the materials presented herein.

Dr. Ashley L. Faulx has no financial or proprietary interest in the materials presented herein.

Dr. Leyla J. Ghazi has no financial or proprietary interest in the materials presented herein.

Dr. Robert E. Glasgow has no financial or proprietary interest in the materials presented herein.

Dr. Eric Goldberg is a consultant for Boston Scientific.

Dr. Fredric D. Gordon has no financial or proprietary interest in the materials presented herein.

Dr. Bruce D. Greenwald has no financial or proprietary interest in the materials presented herein.

Dr. Katarina B. Greer has no financial or proprietary interest in the materials presented herein.

Dr. Kevin Halsey has no financial or proprietary interest in the materials presented herein.

Dr. William R. Hutson has no financial or proprietary interest in the materials presented herein.

Dr. Kimberly Jones has no financial or proprietary interest in the materials presented herein.

Dr. Virendra Joshi has no financial or proprietary interest in the materials presented herein.

Dr. Sergey V. Kantsevoy has no financial or proprietary interest in the materials presented herein.

Dr. Vivek Kaul has no financial or proprietary interest in the materials presented herein.

Dr. Rabi Kundu has no financial or proprietary interest in the materials presented herein.

Dr. Ravinder R. Kurella has no financial or proprietary interest in the materials presented herein.

Dr. Jeffrey Laczek has no financial or proprietary interest in the materials presented herein.

Dr. Robin B. Mendelsohn has no financial or proprietary interest in the materials presented herein.

Dr. James D. Morris has no financial or proprietary interest in the materials presented herein.

Dr. Sean J. Mulvihill has no financial or proprietary interest in the materials presented herein.

Dr. Randall K. Pearson has no financial or proprietary interest in the materials presented herein.

Dr. Douglas Pleskow is a consultant for Boston Scientific.

Dr. Scott Pollack has no financial or proprietary interest in the materials presented herein.

Dr. Darryn Potosky has no financial or proprietary interest in the materials presented herein.

Dr. Waqar A. Qureshi has no financial or proprietary interest in the materials presented herein.

Dr. David A. Schwartz is a consultant for P&G, Abbott, Centocor Ortho Biotech, Salix Pharmaceuticals, UCB, Prometheus, Cellerix, Shire, Axcan. He has received grant support from P&G, Abbott, and UCB.

Dr. Yasser H. Shaib has no financial or proprietary interest in the materials presented herein.

Dr. Brad Shepherd has no financial or proprietary interest in the materials presented herein.

Dr. Andrew Singleton has no financial or proprietary interest in the materials presented herein.

Dr. Colin T. Swales has no financial or proprietary interest in the materials presented herein.

Dr. Caroline R. Tadros has no financial or proprietary interest in the materials presented herein.

Dr. Shyam J. Thakkar has no financial or proprietary interest in the materials presented herein.

Dr. Selvi Thirumurthi has no financial or proprietary interest in the materials presented herein.

Dr. William M. Tierney has no financial or proprietary interest in the materials presented herein.

Dr. Jeffrey L. Tokar has no financial or proprietary interest in the materials presented herein.

Dr. Ryan C. Van Woerkom has no financial or proprietary interest in the materials presented herein.

Dr. Michael J. Walker has no financial or proprietary interest in the materials presented herein.

Dr. Paul E. Wise has no financial or proprietary interest in the materials presented herein.

Dr. Robert C. Wrona has no financial or proprietary interest in the materials presented herein.

INDEX

Printed in the United States
by Baker & Taylor Publisher Services